THE
ULTIMATE GUIDE TO
SELF-HEALING

YOUR PASSPORT TO HEALTH, WELLNESS, AND WHOLENESS

ALLAINE STRICKLEN

THE ULTIMATE GUIDE TO SELF-HEALING
Your Passport to Health, Wellness, and Wholeness

by ALLAINE STRICKLEN

ISBN: 978-0-9858523-1-3

Co-Editors: Allaine Stricklen and Steve Chong
Published by: Steve Chong

Visit: **www.AllaineStricklen.com** for more information on Allaine. For information on bulk orders, permissions, or special requests, contact: **alignwithallaine@gmail.com**

This book is intended to provide general information and practices for personal development, health, and wellness. It is not a substitute for medical advice, diagnosis, or treatment. Readers should consult qualified health professionals regarding any medical conditions or concerns. The author and publisher disclaim any liability arising directly or indirectly from the use of this material.

AUTHOR'S NOTE

Self-inquiry was my first step into the depths of the path of yoga. I have experienced many magical moments—some soaring high, others more challenging. After flying, traveling around the world, and visiting sacred, magnificent places, I've realized it's not the destination that shapes us— **it's the journey and how we choose to respond.**

Through self-inquiry, countless hours of deep meditation and introspection, and even undergoing two brain surgeries, I had a choice to take a deep dive into certain habitual recurring habits and thoughts and as Dr. Joe Dispenza quotes, in his book, *Breaking the Habit of Being Yourself*, I truly understood and embraced this message.

To heal, I surrendered. I let go. I freed myself from the pull of old patterns, limiting beliefs, and the habit of endlessly revisiting the past—whether consciously or unconsciously.

I stopped bulldozing through my triggers and expecting different outcomes and instead began to listen.

As I became deeply uber-aware of my inner dialogue—the subtle stories and habits that were blocking my blessings—space opened. Miracles flowed effortlessly. Purpose was felt in every breath. I realized in that moment that thinking is not the same as feeling, and feeling is where true transformation lives.

I am filled with gratitude for this wisdom. And now, I feel called to share my journey home.

Turning inward, I am healthy. I am whole. I am healed.

Thank you. Thank you. Thank you. And so it is.

My story is ready to be shared.

ALLAINE STRICKLEN'S STORY

Imagine waking up blind and deaf—your world shattered in an instant. That's the nightmare Allaine Stricklen faced, plunging into darkness and silence. But this warrior didn't back down.

Undergoing two grueling brain surgeries back-to-back, she battled through the abyss with unbreakable courage, infinite patience, and sheer willpower. Against all odds, Allaine emerged not just alive, but whole—vibrant, resilient, and ready to roar her story of triumph to the world!

A globally respected Yoga Therapist and Restorative Yoga Master with more than 40 years of experience, Allaine blends deep tradition with the wisdom of her own healing journey. Her mission is bold and uncompromising: to show that yoga meditation is for everyone—no matter your age, shape, injury, or circumstance.

As founder of Gentle Therapeutics Yoga (GTYOGA), she's revolutionized healing with a prop-powered, precision-packed practice rooted in various styles such as Iyengar and Restorative Yoga.

Allaine is an IAYT-certified Yoga Therapist, Yoga

Alliance Master Instructor, and a Certified Scoliosis Specialist trained by icon Elise Browning-Miller. But it's her story of defying the odds, of coming back stronger after blindness and silence, that electrifies audiences and students alike.

From international retreats and teacher trainings to private healing sessions, Allaine's work is more than yoga—it's a testament to human possibility.

Her voice carries the power of someone who has walked through fire and come back to tell the story. And her message is clear: *healing is not just possible, it's your birthright.*

Ignite Your Journey with Allaine's Offerings:

- **Health, Wellness & Personal Healing –** Transform your mind, body, and spirit with tailored strategies designed for helping you to return to balance, harmony and success. Experience personalized guidance through in-person or global online sessions, including one-on-one meditation and healing to ignite your inner strength and spark profound transformation.

- **Retreats & Workshops –** Transform your body, mind, and spirit in breathtaking destinations around the world with immersive programs that combine yoga, meditation, healing practices, and cultural experiences designed to renew and inspire.

- **Gentle Therapeutics Yoga Teacher Trainings –** Master the method and carry the legacy forward with Yoga Alliance–accredited certification programs offering Continuing Education Units (CEUs) for yoga teachers and wellness professionals.

- **Corporate Wellness Programs** – Elevate workplace well-being with customized yoga, meditation, and mindfulness sessions designed to reduce stress, boost focus, and enhance employee health and productivity – in house or online.

- **Restorative & Spinal Health Programs** – Specialized Therapeutics Yoga for scoliosis, spinal conditions, and injury recovery, designed to restore balance, relieve pain, and support long-term healing.

- **Senior & Therapeutic Programs** – Specialized care in chair yoga, Alzheimer's, dementia, and wellness programs for senior centers and facilities.

- **Children & Family Support** – Compassionate coaching for children on the spectrum, including Asperger's and autism, with guidance for families and caregivers.

- **Private Meditation & Healing Sessions –** Unlock inner power with one-on-one guidance.

CONTENTS

THOUGHT IS THE
BEGINNING OF CREATION

INTRODUCTION

Dear Student,

Some time ago, I found myself sitting beneath a palm tree on a quiet island in Australia, waiting for a boat.

I closed my eyes and allowed myself to sink fully into the moment—the gentle breeze of wind, the rhythm of the waves, the earthy scent of the land, and a deep, expansive gratitude for simply being alive. Sitting cross-legged, palms turned upward, I felt a delicate flutter. Opening my eyes, I discovered a butterfly resting gently on my hand. In that instant, something shifted within me.

It was as if the universe had whispered a profound truth: *Just like this butterfly, I too was ready to emerge from my cocoon, to transform from a caterpillar into something free, soaring, and luminous.*

That moment marked the beginning of my own metamorphosis—a journey of healing, self-discovery, and liberation. The three butterflies that grace the cover of this book symbolize the three pivotal milestones of my life, each a testament to resilience, courage, and the deep gratitude that guides me still.

This book is an invitation to you: to embrace your own metamorphosis, to awaken to your unlimited potential, and to step into the freedom and wholeness that have always been within you.

Just as the butterfly takes flight, so too can you.

With **love** and gratitude,

Allaine

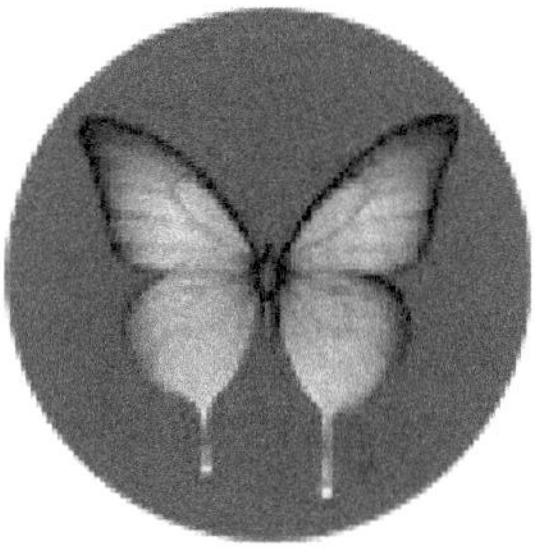

✈ Chapter 1:
AWAKENING YOUR UBER-AWARENESS
Flight 1 – Becoming Your Own Best Healer

🔑 KEY QUESTION / Allaine's Insight

Are you listening to the whispers of your body before it shouts?

🛫 SESSION OVERVIEW

Every great journey begins with awareness, and your healing journey is no different. Your body is always communicating with you. Long before illness or pain arrives, it offers gentle whispers subtle signals of imbalance.

Learning to notice these whispers helps prevent louder disruptions. This session introduces Uber-Awareness—the ability to tune in to the faintest cues of body, mind, and spirit.

By practicing this, you reclaim your power to heal, live with vitality, and move through life with clarity and intention.

KEY TERMS PREVIEW

Before takeoff, familiarize yourself with this essential terminology so you can integrate each practice effectively throughout Flight 1.

- **Uber-Awareness** – Noticing subtle signals from your body, mind, and spirit before they grow into louder disruptions.

- **Journaling** – Recording thoughts, emotions, sensations, and insights to clarify patterns, track progress, and strengthen awareness.

- **Mindful Breathing** – Slow, deep breathing that anchors attention, regulates the nervous system, and calms the mind.

- **Body Scan Meditation** – Progressive awareness from head to toe to notice tension, energy shifts, or areas needing attention.

- **Visualization & Embodiment** – Mentally imagining your body responding with ease and balance; physically feeling and expressing desired outcomes.

- **Mirror Work** – A tool to build self-trust, compassion, and awareness by observing and speaking kindly to yourself in reflection.

- **Micro-Check-Ins** – Brief pauses during the day to observe energy, posture, or emotional state, strengthening ongoing self-awareness.

CORE CONCEPTS

Before takeoff, here are the vital essentials:

- Your body communicates subtle signals before illness or pain emerges.

- Fear constricts; **love** opens the door to healing and connection.

- Presence transforms survival into thriving by aligning you with your body's wisdom.

- Healing is not about fixing what is broken, it's about listening and creating space for balance.

- The brain can rewire itself; small, consistent shifts build lasting resilience in body, mind, and spirit.

▦ DETAILED ITINERARY

Let's explore the chapter's key ideas.

Fear is a natural survival response, but when unchecked, it keeps us trapped in cycles of anxiety, judgment, avoidance, and separation. **Love**, by contrast, opens us to connection, creativity, and healing.

Recognizing when fear drives your thoughts or actions is the first step toward freedom. Awareness is the key to transformation, and transformation begins with noticing. Your body is the most accurate compass you have. Subtle sensations—tightness in the chest, heaviness in mood, or shallow breath—are not random. They are messages calling for attention, compassion, and care.

Noticing signals early allows you to shift your energy before imbalance becomes illness.

🔍 DEEP DIVE: Quiet Signals

Let's look closer at the core insight.

The First Signal - Uber-Awareness is noticing the earliest, most subtle shifts in your body before they grow into louder, disruptive symptoms. This could be faint shoulder tension, a slight change in breathing, or a heaviness in mood.

The more present you become to these whispers, the less your body needs to shout.

Navigating the Inner Skies - Like a pilot adjusting to subtle shifts in wind, you can adjust course when you recognize internal changes. Instead of attaching stress or fear to what you notice, respond with calm presence. This practice strengthens trust in your body's wisdom, allowing greater ease and resilience.

Transforming Awareness into Healing - The

gift of Uber-Awareness is not only prevention but transformation. Meeting your body's whispers with compassion creates space for healing. Awareness shifts you from reacting to creating, from surviving to thriving. Each moment of mindful attention rewires your brain toward resilience and renewal.

Uber-Awareness shows that healing starts in small moments. By noticing early, you learn to trust your body and turn awareness into wisdom.

Key Affirmation:
I honor my body's whispers. Each small signal is wisdom guiding me toward balance, trust, and healing.

⚙ PRACTICAL STEPS TO:
Awaken Your Uber-Awareness

- **Notice Subtle Body Sensations Daily**: Take a few moments each morning to scan your body from head to toe, acknowledging tension, warmth, or ease without judgment.

- **Practice Mindful Breathing:** When stress or tension arises, inhale for 4 counts, exhale for 6. Embrace and use this pause to reset and center yourself.

- **Ask:** *"What message is my body offering me right now?"*: Tune into subtle cues, like slight shifts in posture, heart rate, or energy. Reflect on what your body may be communicating about your needs, emotions, or boundaries.

- **Journal Daily Insights and Take One Honoring Action**: Write down any observations or messages from your body. Choose one small, intentional action to honor what you've learned, reinforcing self-trust.

- **Build Consistency and Notice Patterns**: Track recurring signals or emotional themes over time. Recognize trends, celebrate small victories, and allow awareness to grow into insight and conscious action.

🔔 AWARENESS CHECKPOINTS

Take out your journal and put pen to paper.

- Are you ready to return to yourself and awaken the healer within?

- Where in my life have, I handed over my healing passport?

- How have external influences shaped my plans toward wellness?

- How can I begin trusting my body's navigation system?

- What small readiness checks can I run today to reconnect with my inner healer keeping me more present and uber-aware?

◎ INTENTIONS

By the end of Flight 1, you will:

- Identify where in your life you've given away your healing power or made yourself feel smaller.

- Take introspective moments to observe situations where you surrendered your power by reacting.

- Develop a daily check-in routine to keep your inner healer's communication line clear.

- Embrace curiosity and compassion toward yourself as you explore your inner landscape.

- Cultivate awareness of subtle signals your body sends before discomfort or imbalance arises.

- Practice pausing before reacting to external stressors, maintaining inner calm and clarity.

- Commit to small, consistent daily practices that support holistic self-healing.

- Notice patterns in thoughts, emotions, and bodily sensations to better understand your triggers.

- Strengthen trust in your body's innate wisdom and guidance.

🧰 TOOLS & TECHNIQUES

Here are six practical exercises to strengthen your awareness, rewire limiting patterns, and support your mental, emotional, and physical well-being.

✦ Heart-Centered Listening ✦

Tune into your inner guidance and listen with full presence.

- Find a quiet, comfortable space where you won't be disturbed. Sit with your spine upright yet relaxed.

- Place your left hand over your heart and rest your right hand gently on top.

- Close your eyes and take 5 slow, deep breaths—inhale through your nose, exhale softly through your mouth.

- Allow your breath to settle you into stillness.

- Silently or aloud, ask:
  "What do you want me to know?"

- Listen without rushing, forcing, or judging. Simply allow thoughts, sensations, or images to arise.

- When you feel complete, record every detail—no matter how small—in your journal.

✨ Morning Body Awareness Scan ✨

Check in with your body to notice subtle signals and start your day grounded.

- Upon waking, close your eyes and take 3 slow, grounding breaths, bringing your attention fully into your body.

- Gently scan from head to toe, noticing areas of tension, warmth, tingling, or ease.

- Acknowledge each sensation without trying to change it, simply observing with curiosity and compassion.

- Mentally note any patterns, emotions, or energy shifts, connecting sensations to possible thoughts or intentions for the day.

✦ **Grounding Breath Practice** ✦

Stabilize your nervous system and center your energy.

- Sit or stand with your feet planted firmly on the ground.

- Inhale through your nose for 4 counts, imagining light moving through your body.

- Exhale slowly for 6 counts, sending your energy deep into the earth.

- Repeat 5 times to steady and center your nervous system.

✧ Mirror Work - Reflecting Love ✧

Build self-acceptance and compassion through gentle reflection.

- Stand in front of a mirror in a quiet space. Let your shoulders relax and take a slow, deep breath.

- Look directly into your own eyes. At first, you may feel awkward, shy, or emotional. This is natural.

- Gently say your name, then speak a kind affirmation, such as:
  "[Your Name], *I love you.*"
  "*I am worthy of love and respect.*"
  "*I am proud of the person I am becoming.*" or
  "*I honor my growth every day.*"

- If resistance or self-criticism comes up, notice it without judgment. This is an old pattern ready to be released.

- Stay with yourself for 1–3 minutes, letting the words settle into your heart.

- When ready, smile gently at your reflection and affirm:
  "I am learning to love and accept myself more each day."

- Repeat daily to strengthen self-acceptance and inner support.

✦ Compassionate Journaling

Capture your thoughts and feelings, responding with kindness and insight.

- At the end of your day, write for 5–10 minutes about any signals your body, heart, or mind tried to communicate.

- Reflect on these messages without judgment, honoring what arises with curiosity and compassion.

- Respond to yourself with validation, gratitude, or encouragement, reinforcing inner guidance.

- Identify one intentional action or mindset shift for tomorrow that honors what you've learned today, embedding insight into daily life.

✦ **Daily Gratitude Transmission** ✦

Shift your energy toward rest, receptivity, and positivity before sleep.

- Before bed, note three things you're grateful for—about yourself, your body, or your life.

- Reflect on why each item matters, allowing the feeling of gratitude to deepen and expand.

- Set one positive intention for tomorrow, carrying the energy of appreciation and clarity into your day.

- Take a few slow, grounding breaths to anchor this gratitude and calm your body for restful sleep.

📖 GUIDED PRACTICE:
Emotional Presence and Release

1. Find a quiet, comfortable space where you won't be disturbed. Sit or lie down, letting your body relax.

2. Place your left hand over your heart and your right hand gently on top, creating a sense of grounding and presence.

3. Close your eyes and take three slow, deep breaths—inhale fully, exhale completely—allowing your body and mind to settle.

4. Bring to mind a recurring thought, limiting story, or habitual belief you've noticed. Observe it without judgment.

5. Pause, then gently reframe it with a *"Why"* question affirmation, for example*: **"Why am I finding this easier every day?"** or **"Why am I confident, strong, and energized?"**

6. Visualize the affirmation as a warm, golden light spreading through your body and mind, easing tension and resistance.

7. Repeat the affirmation three times, breathing slowly and noticing any subtle changes in your sensations, energy, or emotions.

8. When ready, open your eyes and briefly journal any insights, sensations, or intentions from the practice.

🧘 MEDITATION SCRIPT:

Guided Meditation for Inner Awareness

Use a slow, calm voice when reading or recording this for yourself or others.

"Close your eyes. Take a few deep breaths, in through the nose, out through the mouth.

Breathe in whatever way feels most natural and comfortable for you—whether that's in and out through the nose, or in through the nose and out through the mouth.

In this masterclass, there's no single 'right' technique; simply follow the rhythm that supports you best. Find your inner still-point.

Bring your attention to your heart and breath. Place your left hand over your heart, your right hand over your lower belly, then connect these centers with uber-awareness.

Feel the gentle rise and fall of your chest and your lower belly - it may help to imagine an extra sets of nostrils in your chest and your belly button.

Watch the expansion of your chest and abdomen several times until you feel calmer and more open, relaxed, and present.

Imagine a warm, golden light shining above you just like the light of the moon or the sunshine.

With each inhale, breathe in healing light. Slowly and steadily, in a continuous stable flow.

With each exhale, release any negative or angry thoughts out into the universe—letting go of doubt, fear, or tension. In other words, primal emotions, fear-based triggers.

Now, ask your inner healer:

'What message do you have for me today?'

Take some time, become still and allow your intuitive inner guidance to shine. Let thoughts, sensations, or images arrive as they come. Trust whatever shows up.

When ready, thank your inner healer, take one deep, grounding breath, and open your eyes.

Taking your time, slowly open your eyes."

🛠 ADDITIONAL TOOLS

Key practices to carry-on into each day to cultivate awareness, presence, and energetic attunement.

- **Check-In:** Place your hand on your heart and ask, ***"What do I need today?"*** Tune into subtle bodily and emotional signals.

- **Evening Reflection:** Journal one whisper, insight, or sensation you noticed during the day, honoring your body's guidance.

- **Gentle Movement:** Stretch or move consciously to release tension and reconnect with your body's natural rhythms.

- **Micro-Pauses:** Take 1–2 minutes to notice your breath, posture, and energy, resetting your presence throughout the day.

- **Mindful Hydration:** Drink water slowly, noticing sensations, temperature, and gratitude for nourishment.

- **Nature Connection:** Observe sights, sounds, and textures outdoors; feel the grounding support of the earth.

- **Protective Visualization:** Imagine a soft light around you, letting in only **love**, peace, and clarity.

- **Digital Boundaries:** Set intentional times to power down devices, disconnect from constant noise, and rest.

😰 REFLECTION PROMPTS

Use these prompts to deepen awareness and guide conscious action.

- Which subtle signals did my body send today that I almost overlooked?

- How did my response support or block alignment?

- How could curiosity and compassion transform these signals into growth?

- What patterns reveal hidden opportunities for change?

- What bold action can I take tomorrow to honor my body's messages?

🛬 LANDING WISDOM:
Trusting Your Inner Compass

Awakening your **Uber-Awareness** is the beginning of your healing path. Each small step of noticing honors your body's wisdom and reclaims your power to heal.

This journey is ongoing—listening, trusting, and living in harmony with yourself.

Conscious attention strengthens your mind-body connection, creating a ripple effect in all areas of life.

Healing is already within you.

Your body is not your enemy, it is your most faithful ally, guiding you toward balance and wholeness.

RECAP OF YOUR JOURNEY

Congratulations — you've completed Flight 1 of your healing journey. Your engines are powered by trust; your coordinates set for transformation.

Keep your navigation tuned to your heart, and remember:

Body right, mind right, spirit ignites— this first flight sets the course for your journey to wholeness.

📝 AFFIRMATIONS FOR FLIGHT 1: Awakening Your Uber-Awareness

Use these positive statements daily to nurture awareness, trust, and healing.

- I listen deeply to my body's signals and honor its wisdom.

- I honor the subtle whispers of my body and respond with care.

- Each small signal from my body guides me toward balance and clarity.

- I trust my body's wisdom and listen with curiosity and compassion.

- I am present, aware, and aligned with my highest well-being.

- My mind, body, and spirit work together to support my health and vitality.

- I release fear and embrace love, healing, and inner guidance.

- I am learning to respond consciously rather than react habitually.

- Every moment of awareness strengthens my inner healer and self-trust.

COMPANION WORKSHEET

COMPANION WORKSHEET

✈ Chapter 2:
REWIRING YOUR STORY

Flight 2 – The Mind as a Portal to Freedom

🔑 KEY QUESTION / Allaine's Insight

What new mental flight paths am I ready to chart, and how will they reshape my health, energy levels, and uber-awareness?

🛫 SESSION OVERVIEW

Welcome aboard Flight 2 of your Self-Healing Masterclass journey. Your thoughts, beliefs, and inner narratives act as your internal flight crew— deeply influencing your biology, behavior, and life experience.

In this session, we'll explore **neuroplasticity**—the brain's natural ability to re-route and upgrade its internal flight paths. You will receive a pre-flight briefing on dissolving limiting beliefs, installing empowering ones, and consciously soaring into new realms of possibility.

KEY TERMS PREVIEW

Keep these essentials in mind to make the most of today's journey.

- **Neuroplasticity** – Your brain can form new pathways, reshaping thoughts, emotions, and habits, allowing you to consciously create lasting change.

- **Law of Resonance** – The energy you hold attracts similar experiences; align your frequency with what you desire to manifest greater harmony, connection, and opportunities.

- **"Why" Question Affirmations** – Ask empowering questions like, ***"Why am I so healthy and strong?"*** to engage your subconscious.

- **Pattern Interruption** – Stop a limiting thought and replace it with one that empowers you.

- **Tesla Method 3-6-9** – Repeat affirmations in structured bursts: 3 morning, 6 midday, 9 evening.

- **Conscious Daily Check-In** – Pause intentionally to notice your mind, body, and emotions. Build Uber-Awareness.

- **Vagus Nerve Reset** – Practices like deep breathing, gentle tapping, humming, or brief cold exposure to calm the nervous system and restore balance.

- **Micro-Pauses & Mindful Presence** – Intentional pauses to notice breath, posture, and energy—stay present.

CORE CONCEPTS

Before takeoff, grasp these essentials:

- Your thoughts and beliefs shape emotions, behaviors, and overall well-being.

- Neuroplasticity lets small, consistent mental shifts reprogram old patterns into empowering new ones.

- Limiting stories create tension and imbalance; awareness lets you notice and redirect, opening space for growth.

- The Law of Resonance amplifies your energy, naturally attracting experiences, people, and opportunities that align with your mindset and intentions.

🗓 DETAILED ITINERARY

Let's map the mind's new flight paths.

Your brain constantly maps reality through internal stories about yourself, others, and the world, shaping your emotions, behaviors, and cellular health.

Outdated narratives can ground your progress, keeping you in stress patterns or dis-ease. Thanks to neuroplasticity, your mind can re-chart its course. Using Law of Resonance and framing affirmations as "Why" questions, you invite curiosity, clarity, and conscious Uber-Awareness.

Example affirmations include:

- ***"Why am I so healthy and strong?"***
- ***"Why am I motivated and energized?"***

Over time, replacing old stories with intentional ones builds calm and peace.

🔍 DEEP DIVE: Uber-Awareness

Let's explore how your mind shapes your reality.

Seeing the Stories You Tell Yourself - Uber-Awareness begins by noticing the subtle mental scripts constantly running in your mind, shaping thoughts, emotions, and actions without conscious review.

Pausing to "listen in" allows you to identify assumptions, limitations, and habitual narratives. Awareness is your first act of sovereignty—reclaiming control of your mental airspace.

Noticing How Beliefs Affect Your Physical State- Every belief triggers physiological responses: brain impulses, hormonal shifts, changes in muscle tone, breath, and heart rate. Uber-awareness invites you to feel these changes.

Examples:

- Self-criticism tenses your shoulders

- Imagining failure makes your breath shallow

- Repeating *"I always fail"* drops your energy

By observing these responses, you illuminate the mind-body connection and decide whether to retire or reroute old beliefs.

Choosing New Flight Paths with Intention - Once you notice old narratives, deliberate re-routing begins. Neuroplasticity supports you: each thought aligned with health, purpose, and joy lays down a new neural pathway.

Key Affirmation:
I am aware of my thoughts and beliefs, and I choose empowering stories that support my body, mind, and spirit.

⚙ PRACTICAL STEPS TO:
Rewire Your Story

- **Log Your Mental Patterns:** Keep a "Mind Journal" for one week. Note moments of stress, doubt, or fear, the story you were telling, and bodily sensations.

- **Pattern Interruption with Law of Resonance Questions:** Replace limiting thoughts with "Why" question affirmations, for example:
"Why am I finding this easier every day?"

- **Introduce a New Narrative into Your Body:** Pair the new story with grounding: hand over heart, slow breath, repeat aloud.

- **Visualize Your New Story, A New Mental Flight Plan:** Imagine living your updated story with confidence, ease, and vitality.

- **Build a Daily Affirmation Checklist**: Write three empowering affirmations to review each morning, setting your mindset for the day.

- **Conscious Daily Check-In**: Pause several times a day to notice your thoughts, emotions, and bodily sensations. Reflect briefly on whether they align with your new story and make small adjustments as needed.

🛎️ AWARENESS CHECKPOINTS

Bring clarity by writing it down.

- Are you willing to awaken deeper awareness and listen to your body's whispers?

- Where in my daily life do I ignore subtle cues from my body and emotions?

- How have patterns of distraction shaped the way I respond to inner signals?

- How can I begin honoring the first signs of imbalance with compassion?

- What simple practices today can help me notice and respond before stress grows louder?

◎ INTENTIONS

By the end of Flight 2, you will:

- Identify hidden limiting internal stories that quietly influence your health and well-being.

- Craft empowering and uplifting "Why" question affirmations to activate the Law of Resonance.

- Practice conscious pattern interruption to rewire old mental pathways, replacing limiting thoughts with empowering alternatives to strengthen new patterns.

- Use visualization and journaling to fully support your new destination.

- Recognize when inherited beliefs or past conditioning shape your choices.

- Strengthen your awareness of subtle self-sabotaging narratives before they take hold.

- Replace disempowering thoughts with language that expands possibility and healing.

- Build a toolkit of mental and emotional practices to redirect your inner dialogue.

- Anchor new beliefs through repetition, self-compassion, and daily mindful awareness over 30 days.

🧰 TOOLS & TECHNIQUES

Here are six practical exercises to strengthen your awareness, rewire limiting patterns, and support your mental and emotional well-being.

✦ Conscious Pattern Interruption & Affirmation Practice ✦

Shift old thought patterns and create empowering mental habits.

- Notice a limiting thought or story as it arises.

- Pause, and replace it with a *"Why"* question affirmation, for example: **"Why am I finding this easier every day?"** or **"Why is it so easy for me to trust the process of life?"** or **"Why am I so confident and resilient?"**

- Allow yourself to feel curiosity as you ask the question, letting your mind explore new possibilities.

- Repeat aloud or silently, letting your mind and body absorb the shift.

- Record insights in a journal to track patterns and progress.

Tesla Method 3-6-9 – Structured Affirmation Reinforcement

Anchor new beliefs through intentional repetition throughout the day.

- Choose one empowering affirmation or "Why" question that resonates deeply with your current goals or intentions.

- Repeat it three times in the morning, six times midday, and nine times before sleep, creating structured moments to reinforce the message throughout the day.

- Pair each repetition with slow, intentional breaths, feeling the affirmation resonate through your body and mind. Notice any subtle shifts in energy or sensation.

- Observe subtle shifts in thought, emotion, and energy. Pay attention to moments when old patterns arise and are gently replaced by this new narrative.

- Reflect briefly after each session, your insights, any resistance, or subtle breakthroughs. These notes help track progress and deepen awareness of how your mind and body respond over time.

- Optional Enhancement: Pair affirmations with visualization—see yourself living fully aligned with the statement. This strengthens neural imprinting and connects mental intention with physical and emotional embodiment.

✨ **Embodied Vision Activation** ✨

Step beyond imagining—live the transformation in your body, mind, and energy.

- Close your eyes and sense the new story you are creating—not just in your mind, but in your posture, breath, and energy.

- Feel how your body moves, your chest opens, and your spine aligns as you step into this version of yourself.

- Anchor the vision with a subtle gesture—hands over heart, arms open, or soft movement—to integrate energy and intention.

- Repeat daily, letting the sensation of embodiment become your inner guide.

Journaling – Mental Flight Logs

Capture your thoughts, emotions, and progress to strengthen awareness.

- Record thoughts, emotions, and experiences each day.

- Note moments of resistance, breakthroughs, or new insights.

- Reflect on patterns, noticing how your mind responds to affirmations and new narratives.

- Use journaling to strengthen conscious awareness and support lasting change.

✦ Vagus Nerve Practices – Calming the System ✦

Activate your body's relaxation response for emotional balance and clarity.

- Engage in slow, deep breathing—inhale through the nose for 4 counts, exhale for 6 counts.

- Hum, chant, or use gentle vocalizations to stimulate relaxation.

- Incorporate slow, mindful movement, such as stretching or yoga.

- Practice daily to enhance receptivity, emotional regulation, and nervous system balance.

✦ Micro-Pauses & Mindful Presence ✦

Check in with yourself and reset attention to the present moment.

- Take intentional breaks to notice posture, breath, and body sensations.

- Observe thoughts and emotions without judgment.

- Reset attention to the present before your next task.

- Notice subtle shifts in energy or mindset during pauses.

- Over time, these micro-pauses strengthen awareness and mental clarity.

📖 GUIDED PRACTICE:
Mental Clarity and Rewiring

1. Find a quiet, comfortable space where you won't be disturbed.

2. Close your eyes and take three slow, deep breaths.

3. Notice a recurring thought or limiting story.

4. Pause and reframe it with a *"Why"* question affirmation, for example:
   "Why am I finding this easier every day?" or
   "Why am I confident and energized?"

5. Visualize the affirmation as golden light spreading through your body and mind.

6. Repeat the affirmation three times, breathing slowly and noticing any shifts in sensation, emotion, or energy.

7. Open your eyes and record any insights, patterns, or new thoughts in your journal.

🎧 AFFIRMATION SCRIPT:

Guided Mind-Body Affirmation Practice

Use a slow, calm voice to anchor your mind, heart, and body in the affirmation.

Find a quiet, comfortable space. Close your eyes and take three slow, deep breaths, allowing your body to settle and your mind to become present.

Bring your chosen *"Why"* question affirmation to mind using the Law of Resonance, for example:

"Why is my body so healthy and strong?"

"Why am I becoming more calm, centered, and resilient each day?"

"Why do I trust my body and mind to guide me wisely?"

"Why am I open to receiving health, clarity, and energy in every moment?"

"Why am I aligned with peace and balance in every moment?"

"Why does love and support flow so easily into my life?"

"Why am I surrounded by opportunities that nurture my growth?"

"Why is my body restoring energy and vitality every day?"

"Why am I safe, supported, and guided in all I do?"

Place your hands gently over your heart and feel the question resonate. Visualize warm, golden energy filling your cells.

Breathe deeply, imagining this energy spreading through your chest, belly, arms, and legs, bringing strength, clarity, and ease.

Repeat your affirmation three times, noticing any images, sensations, or insights that arise.

Pause, then ask your inner guidance:

"What do you want me to know today?"

Receive any messages without judgment.

When ready, take a deep grounding breath, open your eyes, and briefly journal any insights, sensations, or reflections from the practice. Just sit quietly-if drawn to.

🛠️ ADDITIONAL TOOLS

Daily essentials to support awareness and growth.

- **Journaling Rituals:** Write daily reflections on limiting stories and reframe them into affirmations of strength and healing. Over time, this practice reshapes the mental patterns you live by.

- **Mind–Body Check-Ins:** Notice subtle thoughts, sensations, and emotions, and observe how they connect to your inner dialogue.

- **Affirmation Support:** Use audio or digital reminders to anchor empowering beliefs and reinforce your "Why."

- **Visualization Practice:** Dedicate 10 minutes to consciously imagine your new story unfolding with clarity and vitality.

- **Conscious Micro-Pauses:** In everyday routines, pause briefly to reconnect with breath and choose thoughts that align with your healing.

- **Grounding in Nature:** Spend time outdoors to reset, absorb calming energy, and root new narratives in stability.

- **Protective Visualization:** Imagine a golden light surrounding you, clearing old stories and strengthening new ones.

🫥 REFLECTION PROMPTS

Use these prompts to notice patterns and reframe your thoughts.

- What limiting beliefs am I ready to release from my mental carry-on today?

- How do I want to revise my internal roadmap moving forward?

- What emotional turbulence arises as I engage with new affirmations?

- How can I ensure consistency in my self-healing journey?

- Which empowering story can I embody immediately?

🕊️ LANDING WISDOM:
Trusting Your Inner Mind-Body Guidance

Rewiring your story begins with noticing the patterns that shape your thoughts, emotions, and actions. Each moment of awareness is an opportunity to replace limiting narratives with ones that support your health, energy, and clarity.

Small, consistent practices—affirmations, journaling, micro-pauses, and visualization— lay new neural pathways that align your mental landscape with vitality, resilience, and conscious living.

The journey of rewiring your story is ongoing. Each day, you can step into greater freedom, consciously shaping the thoughts, beliefs, and stories that define your life.

RECAP OF YOUR JOURNEY

Congratulations — you've completed Flight 2 of your healing journey. Your mental pathways are strengthened; your inner compass aligned for conscious transformation.

Keep your awareness active and your thoughts intentional, and remember:

Mind clear, beliefs empowered, energy flows—this second flight rewires your story and lays the foundation for lasting health, vitality, and presence.

📝 AFFIRMATIONS FOR FLIGHT 2:

Use these daily to strengthen your mental clarity, cultivate empowering beliefs, and support your inner transformation:

- I notice my thoughts and choose those that empower my health, energy, and clarity.

- Each old story I release makes space for a new, thriving narrative.

- I am capable of rewiring my mind for freedom, joy, and resilience.

- My thoughts create my reality; I direct them with intention and **love**.

- I embrace curiosity, insight, and compassion in every mental shift.

- I am aligned with my highest potential and inner guidance.

- Each day, I strengthen my mental pathways for conscious growth and healing.

COMPANION WORKSHEET

✈ Chapter 3:
LISTENING TO YOUR BODY'S WISDOM

Flight 3 - Tuning Into Your Body

🔑 KEY QUESTION / Allaine's Insight

What signs are your physical body revealing about your inner dialogue?

✈ SESSION OVERVIEW

Welcome to Flight 3 of your Self-Healing journey. Your body is a skilled co-pilot, communicating through feelings, sensations, and subtle energy.

In this session, you'll learn to read your body's signals, understand the intelligence behind symptoms, and develop an empowering inner dialogue.

By gently re-schooling your mind and shifting how you relate to bodily sensations, you strengthen self-trust, deepen awareness, and move toward true wholeness.

KEY TERMS PREVIEW

Before takeoff, familiarize yourself with these essentials so you can integrate each practice effectively throughout Flight 3.

- **Body as Co-Pilot** – Recognizing that your body communicates wisdom, guidance, and intelligence through sensations, tension, and energy shifts.

- **Symptoms as Signals** – Physical discomfort, pain, or fatigue are never random; they reflect unresolved emotions, stress patterns, or energetic imbalances.

- **Emotional Mapping** – Tracing sensations back to their emotional or energetic roots to better understand and respond to the body's messages.

- **Somatic Awareness** – Tuning into body sensations, movement, and breath to deepen the mind-body connection and release tension.

- **Pattern Interruption** – Pausing habitual reactions to bodily signals and replacing fear or judgment with curiosity, care, and conscious response.

CORE CONCEPTS

Key truths for your body-listening journey:

- Your body communicates through sensations, emotions, and subtle energy, guiding your healing.

- Physical symptoms reflect stored emotions, unresolved experiences, and habitual patterns.

- Every sensation is meaningful; tools like body scans, breathwork, somatic meditation, and emotional mapping help translate messages into insight.

- Regular practice strengthens awareness, builds trust with yourself, and opens pathways to health and clarity.

📅 DETAILED ITINERARY

Let's explore the chapter's key ideas.

Too often, we treat symptoms as isolated problems to "fix" rather than messages to understand. Your body never lies—it reflects the totality of your life experience: your thoughts, beliefs, and unprocessed emotions, which surface as pain or discomfort in the physical body.

Pain, tension, fatigue, or discomfort are not random—they're echoes of unprocessed emotional turbulence or energetic blocks. By listening and translating these signals, you can address root causes rather than just managing surface symptoms.

This requires slowing down, tuning inward, and approaching sensations with curiosity, not fear.

🔍 DEEP DIVE: Body Signals

Let's look closer at the core insight.

Noticing Subtle Signals - Uber-awareness is noticing the earliest, smallest shifts in your body and energy before they escalate. This could be a faint tension in your shoulders, a slight change in breathing, or a heaviness in mood. The more you tune in to these whispers, the less your body needs to shout.

Reading the Emotional Map -Every physical sensation carries a story—an emotional or energetic imprint from past experiences. Trace these sensations to their roots with curiosity and compassion. A headache may reveal unspoken resentment; tight hips may hold unprocessed grief. Mapping the emotional origins of your symptoms helps you understand the "why" behind the signals, bridging body, mind, and soul.

Listening and Responding - The body speaks only when it needs to be heard. Pain or discomfort asks, "why did this happen?" Slowing down and tuning into your inner dialogue creates presence. Practices like mirror work, gentle breath inquiry, and tapping open space for honest communication.

By tuning into subtle bodily signals and tracing their emotional roots with curiosity and compassion, you transform discomfort into insight. Consistent awareness and gentle practices create a clear dialogue with your body, strengthening trust, presence, and the path to healing.

Key Affirmation:
I listen deeply to my body's messages, honor its wisdom, and respond with curiosity, compassion, and presence.

⚙ PRACTICAL STEPS TO:
Listen to Your Body's Wisdom

- **Log Track Your Body Signals:** Keep a journal of subtle sensations, moods, or shifts. Ask: **"What might my body be trying to communicate?"**

- **Trace Emotional Roots:** Notice how physical sensations link to past experiences or emotions. For example, tight shoulders may signal unresolved tension. Gently move them up and down to release stress.

- **Create Dialogue:** Use mirror work or gentle tapping to "talk" with your body. Ask questions like, **"What do you need me to know?"** Listen without judgment.

- **Practice Breath Awareness**: Pause during your day and observe your breath. Notice areas of tension and gently release them.

- **Visualize Mind-Body Harmony:** Imagine your body and mind working in alignment, responding calmly to challenges. This visualization strengthens intuitive awareness.

🔔 AWARENESS CHECKPOINTS

Take out your journal and put pen to paper.

- Pause and notice any subtle tension, heaviness, or unusual sensations in your body. *Where is your attention drawn?*

- Name one emotion that might be linked to a physical sensation you feel.

- Take a slow, deep breath and ask your body: *"What do you need me to know right now?"*

- Reflect on a recent minor disruption or stumble—what message might it hold for your growth or awareness?

🎯 INTENTIONS

By the end of Flight 3, you will:

- Notice subtle signals in your body before they escalate into discomfort.

- Track emotions and sensations to uncover the messages behind symptoms.

- Use mirror work, gentle tapping, or breath inquiry to create dialogue with your body.

- Pause to observe how minor disruptions or tension guide awareness and growth.

- Build daily habits of body-listening to strengthen presence and clarity.

- Cultivate curiosity and compassion toward sensations, avoiding judgment.

- Re-school your mind to reframe discomfort into actionable insight.

- Record insights and reflections to deepen self-awareness and guidance.

- Strengthen trust in your body's innate wisdom and its role as co-pilot.

💼 TOOLS & TECHNIQUES

Six practices to tune into your body's signals and deepen self-healing.

✦ Body Scan & Emotional Mapping ✦

Find a quiet, comfortable space where you won't be disturbed.

- Find a quiet space to lie or sit without distraction.

- Take five slow breaths to ground your awareness.

- Move attention from feet to head, noticing sensations without judgment.

- Ask: ***"What is my body trying to tell me?"***

- Breathe into tension or discomfort, creating spaciousness.

- Journal the sensations, emotions, and insights that arise.

✨ Body Awareness Check ✨

Tune in and notice subtle shifts in your body to deepen your mind-body connection.

- Find a quiet space to sit or lie down without interruption.

- Take slow grounding breaths, bringing awareness to your body.

- Gently scan from head to toe, noticing areas of tension or sensation, and observe if any emotions or memories surface.

- Name what you feel (tight, heavy, tingling) without judgment.

- Write down insights to track patterns and grow self-awareness.

✦ Gentle Tapping (EFT) ✦

Rhythmically tap key points to release tension and restore calm.

- Tap gently on meridian points while focusing on the feeling.

- Repeat a phrase like: **"Even though I feel this tension, I deeply accept myself."**

- Notice shifts in sensation or energy.

- Continue until a sense of ease arises.

- Reflect on insights in your journal.

✦ Breath Awareness ✦

A grounding practice to calm the mind and release tension through mindful breathing.

- Pause during your day and observe your natural breath. A grounding practice to release tension, cultivate presence, and strengthen the mind-body connection.

- Find a quiet space where you won't be interrupted. Sit or lie down comfortably and allow your shoulders to relax. Take a few natural, grounding breaths to settle in.

- Pause and observe your natural breathing rhythm. Notice how your chest, belly, and shoulders move with each inhale and exhale.

- Inhale slowly for 4 counts, hold for 2 counts, and exhale for 6 counts. Allow each breath to flow smoothly and gently, without forcing it.

- Scan your body from head to toe, noticing areas of tension, tightness, or discomfort. Breathe into these areas, imagining the breath softening and releasing the tightness.

- Repeat this focused breathing and body scan for 5–10 cycles, maintaining awareness of how your body responds.

- Afterward, pause and notice any changes in sensation, energy, or mood. Journal insights, shifts, or emotions that arose during the practice.

✦ Somatic Movement ✦

Release tension and restore flow through gentle, mindful movement.

- Gently stretch or move your body, noticing sensations.

- Pay attention to areas of tightness or discomfort.

- Move in a way that feels natural, not forced.

- Focus on how movement shifts emotional or energetic blocks.

- Breathe deeply as you explore.

- Journal any insights discovered.

✦ Visualization & Mind-Body Harmony ✦
Cultivate inner balance by visualizing your body and mind in harmony.

- Close your eyes and imagine your body and mind aligned.

- Visualize energy flowing freely through each organ, muscle, and joint, dissolving tension.

- Focus on sensations of ease, calm, and vitality.

- Hold the visualization for several breaths.

- Jot down any guidance, ideas, or sensations that arise.

☐ GUIDED PRACTICE:
Listening to Your Body's Wisdom

1. Find a quiet, comfortable space where you won't be disturbed. Sit or lie down, letting your body relax.

2. Close your eyes and take three slow, deep breaths, settling awareness into your body.

3. Scan your body from head to toe, noticing sensations, tension, or shifts in energy without judgment.

4. Pause at any sensation that stands out and silently ask:
   "What is this message?" or
   "What does my body need me to know?"

5. Use gentle breath awareness, tapping, or light movement to release tension and create space.

6. Visualize energy flowing freely through your body, bringing calm and ease.

7. Open your eyes and journal:
   What messages did your body share?

   Which emotions or insights arose?

   What small step can you take today to honor your body's guidance?

🧘 MEDITATION SCRIPT:

Guided Body Scan for Deep Relaxation

Use a slow, calm voice when reading or recording this for yourself or others.

"Find a comfortable position and gently close your eyes.

Take a slow, deep breath in... and gently exhale.

Again, breathe in deeply... and let the breath out slowly.

Now bring your attention to your feet... notice any sensations—warmth, coolness, tingling, or heaviness.

Simply observe without judgment. Move your attention to your ankles and calves... feel the muscles relax.

Continue to your knees and thighs... notice any tightness or ease, breathing into it.

Bring your focus to your hips and lower back... allow any tension to melt away.

Shift your attention to your belly and chest... feel the rise and fall of your breath.

Now to your shoulders and arms... let them grow heavy and relaxed.

Move to your hands and fingers... notice every subtle sensation.

Bring awareness to your neck and throat... release any tightness.

Finally, focus on your face and head... soften your jaw, relax your eyes and forehead.

Take one more deep breath in... and slowly exhale. When you're ready, gently open your eyes.

Take a moment to notice how your body feels now—lighter, calmer, at ease.

Carry this sense of peace with you as you gently open your eyes and return to the present."

🛠️ ADDITIONAL TOOLS

Everyday practices for body awareness. Return to presence through movement, stillness, and breath—each moment an invitation to truly inhabit yourself.

- Daily body awareness journaling to track subtle sensations and insights.

- Silent meditation or reflective check-ins with your body's wisdom.

- Tapping (EFT) to calm the nervous system.

- Breathwork exercises for tension release and grounding.

- Cushions and blankets for restorative yoga or somatic practices.

- Gentle stretching or movement to release stored tension and improve circulation.

- Nature walks to connect with the body and senses in a grounding environment.

- Mindful hydration—pay attention to sensations and gratitude while drinking water.

🫣 REFLECTION PROMPTS

Use these prompts to notice your body's signals and deepen self-trust.

- What sensation do I notice most often, and what might it be telling me?

- When I feel discomfort, do I ignore it or respond with care?

- How does my body signal stress versus safety?

- What emotions or memories might be linked to what I feel today?

- If my body could speak, what message would it share right now?

✈ LANDING WISDOM:
Tuning Into Your Body's Messages

Your body is wise, always speaking—even in subtle whispers. By noticing sensations, tracing their emotional roots, and responding with curiosity and compassion, you strengthen trust in your innate guidance.

Each moment of mindful attention transforms discomfort into insight, creating a bridge between body, mind, and soul. The more you listen, the more your inner healer can guide you toward balance, clarity, and true wellness.

Your body already holds the answers—you only need to pay attention.

RECAP OF YOUR JOURNEY

Congratulations — you've completed Flight 3 of your healing journey. Your awareness is sharper, and your body's wisdom is now a trusted co-pilot.

Keep your sensors tuned to subtle signals, and remember:

Listen deeply, respond with curiosity, and honor the messages your body shares—*each insight brings you closer to balance, clarity, and self-trust.*

✒️ AFFIRMATIONS FOR FLIGHT 3:
Listening to Your Body's Wisdom

Use these daily to tune in, honor your body's messages, and strengthen self-trust:

- I listen deeply to my body's signals and honor its wisdom.

- Each sensation is meaningful and guides me toward balance.

- I greet discomfort with curiosity, compassion, and presence.

- My body and mind work in harmony to support my healing.

- I trust the messages my body provides and respond with care.

- I am patient and compassionate with myself as I grow in awareness.

- My body is my loyal co-pilot on the journey to **wholeness.**

- I release resistance and allow my body to guide me naturally.

- I honor my body's needs and respond with **love** and attention.

COMPANION WORKSHEET

✈ Chapter 4:
EMOTIONS AS MESSENGERS

Flight 4 – Healing Through Feeling, Beyond Just Thinking

🔑 KEY QUESTION / Allaine's Insight

What is my current emotion trying to convey, and how can I respond with clarity and compassion?

🛫 SESSION OVERVIEW

Welcome aboard Flight 4 of your Self-Healing Masterclass. Emotions are powerful energies in motion—not obstacles to resist.

In this session, you'll learn to embrace emotional waves as guides, transform them into clarity and growth, and deepen connection with your inner self. By feeling emotions fully and without judgment, you restore flow, release stagnation, and open pathways to wholeness and vibrant health.

KEY TERMS PREVIEW

Before takeoff, review these key emotional terms to help you navigate and integrate the practices of Flight 4.

- **Emotional Uber-Awareness -** Recognizing not only surface emotions but subtle nuances beneath, understanding what each feeling communicates.

- **Emotional Mapping** – The process of identifying how emotions connect to bodily sensations, thought patterns, and energetic shifts.

- **Presence with Emotion** – Observing emotions without judgment or attachment, creating space for flow.

- **Emotional Release Practices** – Techniques like conscious breath, gentle sound, and movement to safely release stored energy.

- **Mindful Inquiry** – Asking guiding questions to learn from emotions rather than reacting unconsciously.

CORE CONCEPTS

Before takeoff, here are the vital essentials:

- **Emotions are energy in motion**—signals to be felt, not suppressed.

- **Avoidance creates stagnation**; expression restores flow and balance.

- **Every feeling holds wisdom** about needs, boundaries, or desires.

- **Awareness transforms reaction** into clarity, compassion, and choice.

- **Breath, sound, and movement** are tools to release and reset emotional energy.

📅 DETAILED ITINERARY

Let's explore the chapter's key ideas.

Modern culture often encourages avoidance or numbing of uncomfortable feelings. Yet emotions are natural signals—energies designed to move through you, inform you, and restore balance.

Resisting emotions leads to stagnation, tension, or emotional heaviness. Allowing them to flow—supported by compassion and uber-awareness—softens, shifts, and transforms emotional energy.

Every emotion, whether subtle or intense, carries insight. Discomfort may point to unmet needs, unspoken boundaries, or unacknowledged desires. Joy signals alignment with your authentic self.

🔍 DEEP DIVE: The Language of Emotions

Let's look closer at the core insight.

Witnessing Emotions Without Attachment - Emotions are like clouds drifting across the sky—temporary, ever-changing, not your identity.

Uber-awareness lets you feel fully without getting lost, observing rise and fall naturally.

Using Emotions as Inner Navigation Tools - Rather than suppressing or reacting, ask: ***"What is this feeling trying to show me?"***

Curiosity transforms emotions from obstacles into signals guiding healing steps: setting boundaries, nurturing yourself, releasing old stories, or engaging in movement like yoga or a run.

Emotional Mapping and Flow - Link sensations in the body to emotional and energetic origins. For example: tight shoulders may indicate unexpressed frustration; chest tightness may reveal grief. Breath, gentle sound, or movement helps energy flow and prevents stagnation.

By witnessing emotions without attachment and listening to their messages, you reclaim them as allies instead of adversaries. With uber-awareness, emotions become a compass guiding you toward healing, balance, and deeper self-connection.

Key Affirmation:
I welcome my emotions as wise messengers, allowing their flow to guide me toward healing, clarity, and authentic alignment.

PRACTICAL STEPS TO:
Decoding Emotions as Messengers

- **Track Your Emotions**: Journal each day, noting emotional range. Ask: *"What is this emotion signaling about my needs or desires?"*

- **Trace the Roots**: Explore bodily sensations, thoughts, and energy patterns connected to each feeling. Move or stretch areas of tension to release stuck energy.

- **Witness Without Judgment**: Observe emotions like passing clouds, letting them rise and fall naturally. Simply notice their presence and let them move through.

- **Ask Guiding Questions**: When strong emotions arise, inquire: *"What does this want me to notice or do?"*

- **Use Breath and Movement**: Slow breathing, gentle sighs, or mindful activity help emotions move safely and naturally.

🔔 AWARENESS CHECKPOINTS

Notice the emotions and their messages.

- Am I aware of the emotions that most often trigger me?

- Where do I notice these emotions showing up in my body?

- How can I pause before reacting and create space for choice?

- What truths are revealed when I name my feelings honestly?

- How can I respond with greater awareness instead of old patterns?

🎯 INTENTIONS

By the end of Flight 4, you will:

- Embrace emotions as sacred guides, revealing insight and personal truths.

- Witness feelings fully, without judgment or resistance, allowing natural flow.

- Transform emotional energy into clarity, strength, and inner alignment.

- Cultivate self-compassion, replacing criticism with nurturing presence.

- Deepen mind-body connection through breath, sound, and gentle movement.

- Map emotional patterns to understand unmet needs and unspoken desires.

- Release stagnant energy safely, restoring vibrancy and resilience.

- Record reflections and insights to honor your emotional journey.

- Integrate daily practices that strengthen awareness, presence, and inner guidance.

💼 TOOLS & TECHNIQUES

Six practical exercises to cultivate emotional awareness, release stuck energy, and strengthen your inner guidance.

✦ Emotional Presence Practice ✦

Notice your emotions fully and respond with clarity and compassion.

- Find a quiet, comfortable space where you won't be disturbed. Sit upright yet relaxed.

- Place your left hand over your heart and your right hand gently on top.

- Close your eyes and take 5 slow, deep breaths—inhale through the nose, exhale softly through the mouth.

- Allow your breath to anchor you in the present moment.

- Gently notice any emotions arising. Name them silently or aloud.

- Breathe into the feeling and imagine it moving through you like flowing energy.

- When complete, record observations, insights, or shifts in your journal.

✦ Guided Emotional Release Meditation ✦

Transform emotional energy into insight, clarity, and flow.

- Sit or lie down in a quiet space where you feel supported.

- Close your eyes and take three grounding breaths, bringing awareness to the body.

- Notice an emotion and feel it fully in your body, without judgment.

- On each exhale, sigh, hum, or gently vocalize, allowing the energy to move and release.

- Continue for several cycles, observing subtle shifts in sensation or thought.

- When ready, return attention to your breath and open your eyes.

- Journal the experience, including any insights or patterns that emerged.

✦ **Heart-Centered Journaling** ✦

Capture emotional patterns, messages, and reflections.

- Use your journal daily to track emotions, triggers, and bodily sensations.

- Note insights, questions, or guidance that arise from observing feelings.

- Reflect on how emotions influence thoughts, behaviors, and decisions.

- Write freely without censoring yourself, honoring every observation.

- Record practical steps to respond to emotions with compassion.

✦ Breath and Sound Practices ✦

Use intentional breath and vocalizations to move energy.

- Sit comfortably, hands over heart, and notice areas of tension.

- Inhale slowly and exhale with a sigh, hum, or gentle sound.

- Observe shifts in body, mind, and emotion.

- Combine with gentle stretches to deepen energy flow.

- Journal any insights, patterns, or guidance that arise.

✦ Safe Space Creation ✦

Support emotional exploration with a secure and nurturing environment.

- Select a location where you feel completely safe and supported.

- Use soft lighting, cushions, blankets, or calming objects to enhance comfort.

- Set a clear intention for your emotional practice and honor personal boundaries.

- Minimize distractions to maintain focus and presence.

- Keep your journal, water, or other supportive tools within reach for reflection and ease.

✦ Movement Practices ✦

Release energy, restore flow, and reconnect with your body.

- Engage in gentle yoga, stretching, or mindful walking.

- Focus on areas of tension, observing sensations with awareness.

- Move slowly and intentionally, honoring your body's limits.

- Use breath to support energy flow and emotional release.

- Journal insights, emotional shifts, or guidance that arise during movement.

📖 GUIDED PRACTICE:
Listening to the Message of Emotions

1. Find a quiet, comfortable space where you feel safe and won't be disturbed.

2. Close your eyes and take three slow, deep breaths, noticing the rise and fall of your chest and belly.

3. Bring your attention to a current emotion—name it silently or aloud.

4. Pause and ask a guiding question, such as:
   "What is this feeling trying to show me?" or
   "What message does my heart hold in this moment?"

5. Visualize the emotion as a flowing energy, like a river moving through your body, softening and releasing tension.

6. With each exhale, breathe out resistance or judgment, letting the energy move naturally. Observe shifts in sensation, thought, or insight.

7. Open your eyes and record reflections, patterns, or guidance gained from this emotional practice in your journal.

🧘 **MEDITATION SCRIPT:**

Guided Emotional Flow Meditation

Use a slow, calm voice when reading or recording this for yourself or others.

"Close your eyes and settle into a comfortable, supported position.

Place your hands over your heart and belly if it feels natural.

Take three slow, grounding breaths, noticing the rise and fall of your chest and belly.

Allow your body to soften and your mind to quiet.

Bring your attention to any emotion present. Name it silently or aloud, without judgment.

Simply notice it.

If a thought drifts in, treat it like a passing cloud on a breezy, tranquil day.

With each exhale, sigh, or hum, imagining the energy moving through you, softening, and releasing.

Let it flow naturally, like water returning to the sea.

Observe subtle shifts in your body, mind, or energy.

Allow clarity, lightness, insight, or a deep sense of peace to emerge.

Ask your inner guidance:
'What does this emotion want me to understand?'

Sit in stillness.

Let thoughts or images arrive as they come.
Trust whatever arises.

When ready, thank your inner guidance and
take one more deep, grounding breaths.

Notice any physical sensations, or feelings of
lightness both emotionally and in the body.

Taking your time, slowly open your eyes.

Find deep gratitude in this present moment—
for it is truly a gift."

🛠 ADDITIONAL TOOLS

Key practices to carry-on into each day.

- Journal for daily insights and reflections on emotions, patterns, or messages received.

- Daily emotional and body check-ins: notice subtle sensations, thoughts, and feelings.

- Audio or digital support to reinforce emotional release, breath, or affirmation practices.

- Dedicate 10 minutes for conscious reflection and visualization of emotional clarity and guidance.

- Micro-pauses during routine activities to reconnect with your body, breath, and emotional state.

- Nature connection for grounding, presence, and energy alignment.

- Protective visualization involves imagining a soft, luminous light surrounding you, offering clarity, safety, and compassion.

- Mindful routines can be created by pairing daily actions, such as drinking water or walking, with emotional awareness and gratitude.

REFLECTION PROMPTS

Use these questions to explore your emotions and gain deeper insight.

- What emotions arose today, and how did I respond to them?

- How did noticing and naming these feelings impact my body and mind?

- Which old stories or self-judgments surfaced, and how can I release them?

- What new insights or guidance emerged from observing my emotions?

- What intentional step can I take today to honor and support my emotional journey?

🛬 LANDING WISDOM:
Embracing Your Emotions as Guides

Your emotions are not obstacles—they are powerful messengers offering insight, clarity, and direction. By meeting them with curiosity, compassion, and presence, you transform reactive patterns into balance, resilience, and inner alignment.

Regular practice—through breath, sound, movement, journaling, and mindful awareness—strengthens your emotional fluency and deepens your connection to yourself.

Each day, you can honor your feelings, restore flow, and allow your emotions to guide you toward greater wholeness and vibrant health.

RECAP OF YOUR JOURNEY

Congratulations — you've completed Flight 4 of your Self-Healing Masterclass. You've learned to welcome your emotions as guides, transforming them into insight, clarity, and inner alignment.

Keep your awareness tuned to your heart and body, honoring the messages each feeling carries.

By embracing emotions with curiosity and compassion, you strengthen your resilience, deepen your connection to yourself, and restore natural flow.

📝 AFFIRMATIONS FOR FLIGHT 4:

Use these daily to nurture emotional awareness, compassion, and inner guidance.

- I welcome my emotions as wise messengers, allowing their flow to guide me.

- I observe my feelings without judgment, trusting their guidance.

- Each emotion I feel offers insight into my needs, boundaries, and desires.

- I transform emotional energy into clarity, strength, and alignment.

- I respond to feelings with curiosity, compassion, and conscious choice.

- My mind, body, and heart work together to restore balance and flow.

- I release resistance and allow emotions to move freely and safely.

- I cultivate resilience by embracing emotional wisdom rather than fear.

- Every moment of emotional awareness strengthens my inner healer and self-trust.

✈ Chapter 5:
RELEASING WHAT'S NOT YOURS

Flight 5 – Being in the Here and Now

🔑 KEY QUESTION / Allaine's Insight

How can I recognize when I'm carrying energy that isn't mine—and return my breath, pace, and presence to center?

✈ SESSION OVERVIEW

As energetic beings, we naturally absorb the frequencies of our surroundings, relationships, and our own thoughts. Keeping a state of uber-awareness helps you notice when something you're feeling isn't yours or when your presence has drifted from center.

In this session, you'll learn to recognize and release energetic clutter, ground and protect your energy field, and cultivate mindfulness to stay focused and present. Energy care is not just self-care—it is foundational for deep healing, emotional resilience, and spiritual clarity.

KEY TERMS PREVIEW

Familiarize yourself with these guiding terms before takeoff.

- **Energetic Clutter** – Residual stress, emotions, or energy picked up from others or environments that weigh down your system. This might look like carrying home your coworker's tension after a meeting or feeling drained after being in a crowded space.

- **Grounding** – The practice of reconnecting with your body and the earth to restore stability and presence. Examples include walking barefoot on grass, sitting quietly with both feet on the floor, or taking slow, deep breaths until you feel steady.

- **Clearing** – Releasing stagnant or heavy energy through breath, movement, visualization, or sound. You might sigh deeply, shake out your arms, imagine light washing through your body, or use a mantra to let go of what's not yours.

- **Shielding** – Creating an energetic boundary of light or intention that filters out negativity while allowing **love** and clarity in. This could be picturing a golden bubble around you before entering a stressful situation, or simply affirming, "I am protected and at peace."

- **Mindfulness** – Returning your attention to breath, body, and present moment awareness to stay centered and balanced.

CORE CONCEPTS

Before takeoff, here are the vital essentials:

- You constantly exchange energy with your surroundings; not all energy belongs to you.

- Carrying others' unresolved energy can create fatigue, anxiety, and imbalance.

- Daily energy care practices—grounding, clearing, shielding—nurture vitality.

- Mindfulness keeps you anchored in the present, balancing mind and body.

- Regular energetic hygiene strengthens boundaries and sustains emotional and physical wellbeing.

▦ DETAILED ITINERARY

Let's explore the chapter's key ideas.

Interactions with others, environments, and even your thoughts influence your energetic field. Without intentional clearing and protection, you may absorb negativity, stress, or confusion that isn't yours, creating mental fog, emotional heaviness, or physical fatigue.

Grounding, clearing, and shielding are rituals that restore your natural vitality. Mindfulness techniques engage you in the here and now, preventing accumulation of mental and emotional clutter. Together, these practices maintain clarity, balance, and alignment on your healing journey.

Caring for your energy with this uber-awareness, you create the spaciousness to embody more authenticity in every moment.

🔍 DEEP DIVE: Energy Liberation

Let's look closer at the core insight.

Recognizing What's Not Yours – Jus like stepping into a crowded room and feeling anxious, sometimes the emotions you carry aren't your own. These signals—tension in the chest, mood agitation, or mind fogginess may be absorbed from others. By asking, "Is this mine to carry?" you create space to release what doesn't belong and restore balance.

Grounding and Clearing – Feel the support of the earth in your feet while letting go of stagnant energy, tension, or emotions that no longer serve you. This could look like imagining roots extending from your feet into the earth or visualizing a golden light sweeping away heaviness, restoring clarity and balance.

Shielding and Staying Present - Once you've grounded and cleared, the next step is to protect your field. Picture a luminous bubble of light around you—strong yet permeable— allowing **love**, peace, and joy in, while blocking stress, negativity, and distraction. This shield, combined with mindfulness of breath and body, helps you stay steady and clear even in chaotic environments.

By recognizing what isn't yours, letting go of stagnant energy, and holding your field with care, you reclaim balance and clarity. These practices help your energy flow freely and stay steady in every moment.

Key Affirmation:
I honor my energy, release what does not serve me, and cultivate a protected, clear, and balanced presence.

☼ PRACTICAL STEPS TO:
Maintain Energetic Clarity

- **Ask the Ownership Question:** Pause during your day and ask, *"Is this mine to carry?"* Notice sensations in your body and mind, and visualize releasing any energy that does not belong to you.

- **Ground Daily:** Stand barefoot or sit with your feet on the floor, visualize roots extending into the earth from your soles, and take slow breaths to connect yourself and restore stability.

- **Clear Your Field:** Use conscious breath, gentle sound, or guided visualization to release stagnant, heavy, or stuck energy, allowing tension, mental fog, or emotional fatigue to dissolve and restore clarity.

- **Stay Present:** Return attention to your body, breath, and surroundings whenever you feel off-center to remain grounded in the present.

- **Protect Your Space:** Imagine a light-filled boundary that allows positivity in while blocking stress or negativity, reinforcing it before entering busy or charged environments.

- •**Daily Energy Check-In:** Take brief moments to notice tension, heaviness, or agitation and use grounding, clearing, or shielding as needed to stay balanced.

🔔 AWARENESS CHECKPOINTS

Open your journal and note your observations about energy and presence.

- When do I notice I am carrying energy that isn't mine?

- Which sensations in my body signal absorbed tension or fatigue?

- How can I release what doesn't belong to me without resistance?

- What grounding or clearing practices bring me back to center most effectively?

- How can I protect my energy and stay present throughout the day?

🎯 INTENTIONS

By the end of Flight 5, you will:

- Identify moments when you are carrying energy that isn't yours and create space to release it.

- Observe and understand subtle signals in your body that indicate energetic imbalance or tension.

- Develop consistent grounding, clearing, and shielding routines to maintain energetic clarity.

- Cultivate mindful presence, responding to stress or external influences with calm and awareness.

- Strengthen trust in your body's innate wisdom to guide your energy, choices, and healing journey.

- Commit to daily practices that protect and nurture your energetic, emotional, and mental well-being.

- Recognize patterns in absorbed energy, emotions, and reactions to prevent fatigue and maintain balance.

- Embrace curiosity and compassion toward yourself as you navigate energetic self-care.

- Integrate awareness of your energy field into all areas of life, fostering clarity, vitality, and inner harmony.

🧰 TOOLS & TECHNIQUES

Here are six practical exercises to release what isn't yours, protect your energy, and stay grounded, clear, and present.

✦ Energetic Ownership Check-In ✦

Tune into your energy field and notice what belongs to you.

- Find a quiet space where you won't be disturbed.

- Sit or stand with a grounded posture, feet firmly on the floor.

- Close your eyes and take three slow, deep breaths, feeling the rise and fall of your chest and abdomen.

- Gently ask:
  "Is this mine to carry?"

- Observe any tension, heaviness, or agitation in your body or mind.

- Visualize exhaling or sweeping away energy that isn't yours, allowing clarity and balance to return.

- Spend a few moments noticing how your body and mind feel once you've released what doesn't belong.

- Journal any insights or observations about external energies that often affect you.

✦ Grounding and Earth Connection ✦

Anchor yourself to the earth to restore stability and presence.

- Stand or sit with your feet on the floor, imagining roots growing into the earth.

- Breathe slowly, drawing calm and stability upward from the ground.

- Notice sensations of support, heaviness, or steadiness in your body.

- Add gentle stretches or mindful movements to deepen the connection.

- Use daily, especially when feeling scattered or drained, to restore balance, and reconnect with your inner stability.

✦ Energetic Clearing Practice ✦

Release stagnant, heavy, or misaligned energy from your body and field.

- Find a quiet, comfortable space where you won't be disturbed.

- Sit or stand with a grounded posture, feet firmly on the floor.

- Close your eyes and take three slow, deep breaths, feeling your energy settle into your body.

- Visualize your personal energy field surrounding you — like a gentle glow or subtle vibration.

- Bring to mind any person, place, or situation that feels heavy or intrusive.

- Gently ask:
  "Is this mine to carry?" and
  "Does this energy serve my highest good?"

- If the answer feels like *no*, exhale or sweep your hands downward, releasing the energy from your field.

- Imagine a soft light — gold, white, or violet — filling the space you've just cleared, restoring calm, clarity, and wholeness.

- Spend a few moments noticing the difference in how your body and mind feel once you've reclaimed your energy.

- Journal any insights, sensations, or recurring themes you observe.

✦ **Protective Shield Visualization** ✦

Strengthen your energetic boundaries and maintain presence in chaotic spaces.

- Visualize a luminous, permeable bubble surrounding your body beyond your physical form.

- Affirm it allows **love**, peace, and joy in while keeping negativity and draining energy out.

- Practice before entering crowded, stressful, or emotionally charged spaces.

- Combine with grounding practices to enhance stability, presence and calm.

- Notice how your energy feels afterward, observing clarity and centeredness.

✦ Energy Clearing Through Writing ✦

Release what doesn't belong to you by giving it a place outside your body and mind.

- Take a blank page and write down thoughts, emotions, or burdens that feel heavy or not truly yours.

- Don't censor — let the words flow freely, even if they don't make full sense.

- Once complete, read it silently and acknowledge:
  "This is not mine to carry."

- Tear, crumple, or safely burn the page as a symbolic release.

- Close with three deep breaths.

✦ End-of-Day Reflection and Release ✦

Close your day with awareness and energetic reset.

- Sit quietly and place your hands over your heart, bringing attention to your body and breath.

- Review moments from the day where your energy felt scattered or heavy.

- Visualize releasing anything that doesn't belong to you, letting it dissolve away.

- Reflect on subtle shifts, sensations, or insights that arose during this practice.

- Journal your observations and set a clear intention for a grounded, centered, and balanced tomorrow.

📖 GUIDED PRACTICE:
Releasing What's Not Yours

1. Find a quiet, comfortable space where you can sit or lie down undisturbed.

2. Close your eyes and take three deep, grounding breaths, softening your shoulders and jaw.

3. Visualize any heavy or stagnant energy in your body as a mist, cloud, or color that does not belong to you.

4. On each exhale, release this energy out through your breath, your skin, or down through your roots into the earth for cleansing.

5. Imagine a gentle stream of light washing over you, clearing away all that is not yours and restoring your natural radiance.

6. Affirm silently or aloud: *"I release what is not mine. I return to myself, whole and free."*

7. Rest for a moment in this clear space, then slowly open your eyes, carrying lightness and clarity into the rest of your day.

🧘 MEDITATION SCRIPT:

The Practice of Energetic Release

Use a slow, calm voice when reading or recording this for yourself or others.

"Find a comfortable position, either sitting or lying down.

Close your eyes and take three gentle, steady breaths, arriving fully in this moment.

Bring your awareness to your body. Notice any weight you may be carrying—emotions, expectations, or thoughts that do not truly belong to you.

Without judgment, simply acknowledge what feels heavy, foreign, misaligned, or may have triggered you.

With each exhale, imagine these energies leaving you, like smoke dissolving into the air or leaves carried away by a gentle stream.

You don't need to hold them. You don't need to carry them.

Let them go with ease.

Refocus your attention on what you do want.

Now, breathe in deeply and imagine drawing in what is truly yours—your peace, your clarity, your vitality.

Feel it filling your body, filling your whole body, mind, and spirit.

Envision yourself surrounded by a soft, luminous field of light.

This field strengthens your connection to what is authentic, while allowing all that is not yours to pass by without entering.

It is a feeling of safety and protection.

Silently affirm:

'I release what is not mine. I return to my own center. I am clear, whole, and free.'

Take a few more breaths, allowing this sense of release and clarity to settle into your being.

When ready, gently open your eyes, carrying this lightness and inner freedom with you into the rest of your day."

🛠️ ADDITIONAL TOOLS

Daily practices to support energetic clarity and presence.

- **Morning Grounding:** place your feet on the floor, visualize roots into the earth, and ask,
  "What energy do I need to carry today?"

- **Evening Reflection:** journal one moment where you noticed energy that wasn't yours and how you released it.

- **Embodied Release Practices:** Explore deeper movement such as shaking, flowing stretches, or gentle yoga to clear stagnant energy and restore balance. Notice how energy shifts as you move.

- **Energetic Micro-Pauses:** Upgrade your pauses into full resets — take 2 minutes to breathe, visualize releasing any heaviness, and consciously invite lightness back into your field.

- **Conscious Hydration:** As you drink water, hold the intention that each sip cleanses old energy and nourishes vitality. Speak an affirmation silently or aloud, such as:
  "I receive clarity with every breath and sip."

- **Nature as a Mirror:** Go beyond walking barefoot — let nature teach you. Notice how trees release leaves, rivers keep flowing, or the wind clears the air, and reflect on how you can embody the same wisdom.

😨 REFLECTION PROMPTS

Use these prompts to deepen awareness and guide conscious action.

- When do I feel cluttered, heavy, or drained, low in energy?

- Which grounding or shielding practices restore my balance most effectively?

- How does mindfulness of breath, body, and energy help me stay present and clear?

- What shifts do I notice in my energy, presence, or mood do I notice?

- What daily intentions support my energetic clarity and safety?

🛬 LANDING WISDOM:
Carrying What No Longer Serves You

As you come to the close of this flight, remember that not every weight you feel belongs to you.

Life constantly offers you opportunities to notice—*"Is this mine, or have I picked up what's not mine to carry?"* That single moment of awareness creates freedom.

Releasing is not avoidance—it is clarity. When you ground, clear, and shield, you return to your calm center. From here, you can meet life with compassion and resilience, without losing yourself.

True presence arises not from holding everything, but from letting go of what is not yours.

RECAP OF YOUR JOURNEY

Congratulations — you've completed Flight 5 of your healing journey. You've learned to protect your energy, clear what doesn't belong, and ground yourself in strength. Each moment of uber-awareness strengthens your ability to walk through life with clarity and confidence.

Keep your shield of awareness polished and remember:

Energy guarded, clarity restored, spirit free—this flight shows your inner power so you can move forward with lightness, resilience, and trust in the path ahead.

📝 AFFIRMATIONS FOR FLIGHT 5:
Releasing What's Not Yours

Use these statements daily to nurture energetic clarity, presence, and protection.

- I recognize when energy does not belong to me and release it with ease.

- I honor my body's subtle signals and respond with care and awareness.

- I am grounded, clear, and fully present in each moment.

- I protect my energy while allowing **love**, joy, and peace to flow in.

- I cultivate inner calm, clarity, and resilience throughout my day.

- I trust my body and intuition to guide my energetic boundaries.

- I release tension, heaviness, and absorbed energy with gentle intention.

- I move through the world centered, aligned, and energetically whole.

- Each moment of awareness strengthens my inner healer and self-trust.

COMPANION WORKSHEET

COMPANION WORKSHEET

✈ Chapter 6:
THE HEART'S TRUE COMPASS

Flight 6 – Navigating From Fear to Love

🔑 KEY QUESTION / Allaine's Insight

How do I deepen my über-awareness to recognize when I am operating from fear versus **love**, limitation versus expansion, or negativity versus positivity?

✈ SESSION OVERVIEW

At the heart of healing lies a fundamental choice: to operate from **love** or fear—the power state versus the primal state.

This session teaches you to identify fear-based patterns, consciously shift toward **love**, and cultivate self-acceptance, emotional resilience, and healing potential. By choosing **love** as your guiding frequency, you harmonize mind, body, and spirit, laying the foundation for lasting transformation.

KEY TERMS PREVIEW

Familiarize yourself with these guiding terms before takeoff.

- **Fear** – A primal survival response that manifests as contraction, resistance, limiting beliefs, self-doubt, blame, shame, or painful disconnection. Fear narrows perception and restricts vitality, creativity, and authentic emotional flexibility.

- **Love** – An expansive, heart-centered frequency that nurtures trust, radical self-acceptance, genuine connection, and conscious transformation. Love opens pathways for profound healing, resilience, and lasting personal growth and freedom.

- **Fear-Based Patterns** – Habitual thoughts, behaviors, or emotions rooted in fear rather than choice. They often repeat in relationships, work, or daily decisions.

- **Love-Based Responses** – Intentional actions, thoughts, and feelings that arise from presence and the heart's frequency, nurturing clarity, compassion, and growth.

- **Conscious Shift** – Noticing fear, pausing, and choosing **love** through awareness, breath, affirmations, or visualization.

- **Heart-Centered Awareness** – Tuning into the body, breath, and emotions to gently and wisely guide decisions from **love** rather than fear.

CORE CONCEPTS

Before takeoff, here are the vital essentials:

- Fear and love are opposing energetic frequencies shaping perception, decisions, and lived experience.

- Fear contracts—appearing as resistance, judgment, self-doubt, and disconnection; **love** expands, inviting trust, acceptance, and healing.

- Recognizing fear-based patterns consistently creates openings for conscious choice and transformation.

- Repeatedly choosing **love** rewires the nervous system, deepens resilience, and harmonizes mind, body, and spirit.

▦ DETAILED ITINERARY

Let's explore the chapter's key ideas.

Fear is a primal survival response, but when unexamined, it narrows perception, restricts creativity, and keeps us trapped in self-doubt, judgment, and disconnection. **Love**, in contrast, is expansive—inviting trust, radical self-acceptance, and deeper connection with self and others.

Developing uber-awareness allows you to notice subtle fear signals—tight shoulders, racing thoughts, shallow breathing—before they escalate. Observing fear without judgment opens space to consciously choose love. Pausing, breathing, and bringing attention to the heart center rewires responses. Gratitude, reflection, and mindful presence reinforce love as your default frequency.

🔍 DEEP DIVE: Energy Shifts

Let's look closer at the core insight.

Recognizing Fear Currents - Fear flows subtly through body and mind before we notice it. Tight shoulders, racing thoughts, shallow breath, or a sense of heaviness are early warning signs. These currents narrow perception, contract energy, and trigger reactive patterns. Tuning into these signals gives you the opportunity to respond consciously rather than react unconsciously.

Tuning into Love Waves - Love moves with a gentle, expansive rhythm, inviting trust, openness, and connection. Unlike fear, which contracts and isolates, love encourages flow and flexibility. When you intentionally shift attention to the heart, breathe with presence, or practice gratitude, you activate these waves. Over time, these waves become the natural current guiding all your decisions.

Navigating Subtle Tides - Life constantly moves between fear and **love**; subtle tides rise and fall within every moment. By cultivating heart-centered awareness, you can sense these shifts early, step back, and choose your response. Recognizing the ebb and flow of emotional energy allows you to ride challenges gracefully, transforming fear-driven reactions into intentional, love-based choices.

By noticing the subtle currents of fear and the gentle waves of **love**, you gain the power to consciously choose your response in every moment. It's time to let **love** guide your energy, decisions, and relationships.

Key Affirmation:
I notice the shifts within me and choose love as my guiding current.

⚙ PRACTICAL STEPS TO:
Shifting From Fear to Love

- **Spot Fear Early –** Throughout the day, notice subtle signals such as a racing heart, clenched jaw, tight shoulders, or looping thoughts. Recognize these as gentle alerts rather than threats.

- **Step Back and Observe –** Watch fear's narrative with compassion and curiosity. Avoid judgment, and remind yourself that noticing is the first step toward conscious choice.

- **Pause and Breathe –** Take a deliberate breath, inhaling for 4 counts and exhaling for 6. Use this moment to create space and align with **love**.

- **Feel the Shift in Your Body** – Notice tension releasing, breath softening, and mental clarity emerging as you intentionally choose **love**.

- **Practice Daily Gratitude** – Identify three things you appreciate in the moment. Gratitude tunes your heart, reinforces **love's** frequency, and strengthens resilience.

🔔 AWARENESS CHECKPOINTS

Tune in, reflect, and capture your inner shifts.

- Notice early signals of fear in your body, such as tight shoulders, racing heart, or shallow breath.

- Observe your thoughts and emotional patterns without judgment, identifying when fear is influencing decisions.

- Tune into subtle shifts in energy—does it feel constricted, heavy, or expansive and open?

- Reflect daily on moments when you aligned with **love** versus fear, and celebrate small shifts toward heart-centered awareness.

⊙ INTENTIONS

By the end of Flight 6, you will:

- Identify moments when fear has influenced your thoughts, emotions, or decisions.

- Observe situations where you reacted from contraction rather than heart-centered awareness.

- Develop a daily check-in practice to sense subtle fear signals in your body and mind.

- Approach your inner experiences with curiosity and compassion, noticing both fear and **love**.

- Cultivate awareness of bodily sensations, energy shifts, and emotional cues before tension escalates.

- Practice pausing and breathing before responding, allowing love to guide your actions.

- Commit to small, consistent practices that strengthen your alignment with **love's** frequency.

- Track recurring patterns of fear and **love** to deepen self-understanding and conscious choice.

- Strengthen trust in your heart's guidance and the wisdom of your body's subtle signals.

💼 TOOLS & TECHNIQUES

Here are six practical exercises to strengthen your awareness, shift from fear to love, and support your emotional, mental, and physical well-being.

✦ Identifying Fear Triggers ✦

Notice subtle signals in your body and mind that indicate fear.

- Find a quiet, undisturbed space where you can sit or lie down comfortably. Let your spine be naturally upright, relaxed but alert.

- Close your eyes and take five long, slow, intentional breaths. With each exhale, release any surface-level tension. Let yourself settle.

- Begin to observe. Are there areas of tightness in your body—your chest, jaw, belly, shoulders? Is your breath shallow or restricted? Do your thoughts feel rushed, circular, or protective?

- Stay curious, not judgmental. These are signals—not problems. What emotions or memories arise alongside these sensations? What are you defending against or trying to avoid?

- Reflect: What do these signals tell you about your fears? Are they tied to past experiences, unmet needs, or habitual beliefs? What reactions tend to follow these triggers in daily life?

✦ Check-In Accountability ✦

*Track your moments of fear and **love** throughout the day.*

- At any pause, ask: *"Where did I operate from **love**? Where did fear show up?"* and notice the subtle shifts in your energy.

- Journal your reflections without judgment, recording both internal sensations and external reactions.

- Notice patterns or triggers and consider small ways to respond differently, more positively next time.

- Reflect on how choosing love over fear affected your interactions, decisions, or mood.

✨ Gratitude Practices ✨

*Tune your heart toward **love** and resilience.*

- Each day, take a few intentional moments to name three things you are grateful for—these can relate to yourself, your relationships, your body, or the world around you.

- Be specific and notice the feelings that arise as you reflect.

- Express your gratitude outwardly when possible, whether through a kind note, a gentle word, or a silent acknowledgment to others.

- Allow the energy of your appreciation to ripple beyond yourself, strengthening connection and positivity.

- Pause fully to feel gratitude in your body—notice warmth in the chest, a softening in tension, or a sense of lightness.

- Let this practice shift your energy from fear or contraction to **love** and receptivity.

- Place your left hand on your heart, right hand over it. Gently rub three clockwise circles, imagining white light soaking into your heart and soul. Then shake off your hands—3, 6, or 9 times—like flicking off old energy.

- Over time, journaling and daily acknowledgment of gratitude deepen awareness, cultivate joy, and anchor **love** as your guiding frequency.

✦ Love Anchoring Visualization ✦

*Reinforce your alignment with **love** and stabilize your energy throughout the day.*

- Sit or lie comfortably in a quiet space, spine relaxed, eyes closed.

- Take 5 deep, slow breaths.

- Visualize a radiant light expanding from your heart, flowing through your body, dissolving tension and fear.

- Silently repeat: *"I am guided by **love**. Fear flows away, and I am safe and supported."*

- Imagine this light connecting to your surroundings, sending warmth and compassion outward.

✦ Heart Resonance Mapping ✦

*Map your body's response to fear and **love** to strengthen awareness and conscious choice.*

- Sit comfortably and place your hands lightly over your heart and solar plexus.

- Recall a recent moment of fear—notice where it shows up in your body. Observe sensations without judgment.

- Shift attention to a moment of **love**, trust, or gratitude. Observe the warmth or expansion.

- Compare how fear contracts and **love** expands.

- Journal your notes to build a personal body map and spot fear early.

✦ Love Infusion Breath ✦

Transform subtle fear signals into heart-centered energy using conscious breath.

- Sit or stand with a straight, relaxed spine and hands resting on your heart.

- Inhale deeply through the nose for 4 counts, filling your chest with light.

- Hold for 2 counts, feeling the energy expand. Exhale through the mouth for 6 counts, releasing fear and tension.

- Repeat 5–7 cycles, each time feeling your heart expand and your mind calm.

- End by silently affirming: *"I breathe in love, I release fear. My heart guides every choice."*

⬜ GUIDED PRACTICE:
Choosing Love in the Moment

1. **Find Your Quiet Space** – Sit or lie comfortably in a place where you won't be disturbed. Keep your spine upright yet relaxed.

2. **Anchor Your Awareness in the Heart** – Place your left hand over your heart, right hand gently on top. Close your eyes and take 5 slow, deep breaths.

3. **Scan for Fear** – Notice any tension, racing thoughts, tightness, or heaviness in your body. Acknowledge these sensations without judgment, they are signals, not threats.

4. **Pause and Breathe into Love** – Inhale for 4 counts, exhale for 6. Visualize warm, radiant light expanding from your heart, dissolving tension and fear.

5. **Affirm Your Choice** – Silently or aloud repeat: *"I choose love over fear. I am safe, supported, and open to guidance."*

6. **Observe the Shift** – Notice the body relaxing, breath softening, and mind calming. Feel the subtle expansion of energy as **love** replaces contraction.

7. **Close with Reflection** – Gently open your eyes. Journal any insights, sensations, or lessons. Identify one conscious action to respond with **love** in the next situation you encounter.

🧘 MEDITATION SCRIPT:

Guided Meditation for Centering in Love

Use a slow, calm voice when reading or recording this for yourself or others.

"Close your eyes. Bring your attention to your heart.

Feel the gentle rise and fall of your chest and your lower belly.

Imagine your breath flowing as if through an extra set of nostrils in your chest and belly.

Notice any tension, tightness, or subtle signals of fear without judgment.

Watch your chest and abdomen expand and soften several times until you feel calmer, more open, and present.

Visualize a warm, radiant light glowing from your heart—like the sun or the moon, steady and comforting.

With each inhale, draw this loving light into your body. With each exhale, release fear, doubt, and tension, letting them dissolve into the universe.

Silently ask:
'What message does my heart have for me today?'

Remain still. Allow thoughts, sensations, or images to appear naturally.

Perhaps you are drawn to picking up your journal and pen of choice and recording any relevant wisdom for you to contemplate.

Sometimes if I simply notice my internal dialogue and simply refocus on a different outcome.

Trust whatever shows up without forcing it.

Remember to attract, not chase what you want. Be specific with exactly what you desire or wish for.

You will see immediate results.

When ready, thank your heart and inner guidance, take one or two grounding deep breaths, and gently open your eyes."

🛠 ADDITIONAL TOOLS

Key practices to strengthen your heart-centered awareness.

- **Morning Heart Alignment:** Begin with your hand over your heart, and instead of only noticing fear, set a loving intention:

  "Today, I choose to meet challenges with compassion and clarity."

  Feel your heartbeat as a rhythm of trust.

- **Evening Heart Reflection:** Journal not only a fear-based moment and a loving choice, but also how your heart felt in each. This helps you recognize the embodied difference between contraction and expansion.

- **Embodied Heart-Opening:** Incorporate gentle, flowing movements such as chest-openers, side stretches, or heart-centered yoga postures. Move with breath to release tension and invite openness.

- **Heart-Centered Micro-Pauses:** Take 1–2 minutes throughout the day to place your awareness in your heart space. With each breath, subtle energy shifts and return to your inner compass of **love**.

- **Nature Protective Heart Visualization:** Envision a radiant, pulsating light surrounding your body, centered in your heart. With each inhale, it grows stronger, allowing in **love**, peace, and trust while dissolving fear at the edges.

😟 REFLECTION PROMPTS

Use these prompts to notice fear, anchor **love***, and cultivate heart-centered awareness.*

- When does fear appear in thoughts, feelings, or actions?

- How does choosing **love** change your experience?

- How can you bring more **love** into daily interactions?

- What one action can respond to fear with **love** today?

- How does gratitude shift your energy and perspective?

🕊 LANDING WISDOM:
Listening to Your Heart

Remember, choosing **love** over fear is the cornerstone of your healing and growth. Each moment you notice fear and consciously shift to **love** strengthens your inner guidance and expands your emotional resilience.

This practice is ongoing—pausing, observing, and responding with heart-centered awareness cultivates harmony within yourself and in your relationships. **Love** is already within you.

Your heart and body are allies, offering constant guidance. By trusting these signals, you align with your true self, transforming fear into freedom and creating a foundation for lasting peace, connection, and wholeness.

RECAP OF YOUR JOURNEY

Congratulations — you've completed Flight 6, navigating from fear to **love**. Your inner compass is attuned, and your heart-centered awareness is stronger with each conscious choice.

Keep your attention tuned to subtle signals of fear and **love**, and remember:

Fear noticed, **love** chosen, heart opens— each shift strengthens your resilience and deepens your connection to yourself and the world.

📝 AFFIRMATIONS FOR FLIGHT 6:
Listening to Heart Signals

*Use these daily to strengthen your heart-centered awareness, shift from fear to **love**.*

- I listen deeply to my body's signals and honor its wisdom.

- I honor the subtle whispers of my body and respond with care.

- Each small signal from my body guides me toward balance and clarity.

- I trust my body's wisdom and listen with curiosity and compassion.

- I am present, aware, and aligned with my highest well-being.

- My mind, body, and spirit work together to support my health and vitality.

- I release fear and embrace **love**, healing, and inner guidance.

- I am learning to respond consciously rather than react habitually.

- Every moment of awareness strengthens my inner healer and self-trust.

COMPANION WORKSHEET

COMPANION WORKSHEET

✈ Chapter 7:
THE ART OF LETTING GO

Flight 7 – Releasing Energetic Baggage and Creating Space

🔑 KEY QUESTION / Allaine's Insight

What past pain, stories, or resentments am I still holding onto?

🛫 SESSION OVERVIEW

First, we must clearly identify what we want—*only then can we let it go*. Letting go is a sacred, active step in your healing journey. This chapter guides you through releasing past pain, stories, and resentments that weigh down your energy and keep you stuck in old patterns.

You'll learn rituals and daily practices that free your emotional and energetic space, inviting your highest potential to emerge. By consciously releasing these burdens, you create an inner environment where healing, joy, and new possibilities can flourish.

✳ KEY TERMS PREVIEW

Familiarize yourself with these guiding terms before takeoff:

- **Identifying Energetic Baggage –** Emotional, mental, or spiritual weight carried from past experiences, stories, or resentments that limit freedom and clarity.

- **Letting Go –** The intentional practice of releasing what no longer serves you, freeing space for healing, growth, and joy.

- **Forgiveness –** Choosing compassion and understanding toward yourself or others, not condoning harm, but reclaiming personal power and peace.

- **Release Visualization –** A focused mental exercise where you imagine carrying, setting down, or dissolving emotional or energetic weight, creating space for healing, clarity, and new opportunities.

- **Physical Decluttering –** Organizing or releasing items in your environment to mirror and support internal emotional and energetic clearing.

- **Inner Alignment –** The state of harmony between thoughts, emotions, and actions, achieved by consciously releasing what weighs you down.

💡 CORE CONCEPTS

Before takeoff, here are the vital essentials:

- Holding onto pain, resentment, and old stories keeps you anchored in the past.

- *Letting go* is an empowered, intentional practice—not passive forgetting.

- Forgiveness and release create energetic space for healing and growth.

- Physical decluttering supports emotional and energetic clearing.

- Daily movement practices—running, yoga, martial arts—cultivate freedom and new beginnings.

📅 DETAILED ITINERARY

Let's explore the chapter's key ideas.

Emotional and energetic baggage often shows up as heaviness, fatigue, or recurring challenges. True healing requires actively recognizing and releasing these burdens to move forward with freedom, clarity, and purpose.

Letting go doesn't mean condoning harm or denying feelings; it means consciously choosing not to carry past weight into your present or future.

Old stories or resentments act like heavy anchors, appearing as emotional triggers, tension, or stagnation. Intentional mindful practices remove these anchors, restore energy flow, and cultivate lightness and sustainable growth.

🔍 DEEP DIVE: Anchor Clearing

Let's look closer at the core insight.

Recognizing What We Carry - Much of our emotional baggage is unconscious, showing up as repetitive thoughts, emotional triggers, or physical tension. Identify stories, resentments, or expectations that weigh on your mind, body, or spirit. Awareness is the first step to intentional release. By naming what you carry, you reclaim the power to choose freedom over habitual patterns.

The Energy of Letting Go - Releasing old anchors shifts your internal frequency, creating space for clarity, joy, and renewed resilience. Emotional release isn't about forgetting or denying—it's about mindfully redirecting energy from stagnation into forward movement.

Embodying Lightness and Flow - As you shed old stories, notice the subtle changes in posture, breath, and emotional tone. Lightness doesn't arrive instantly, but daily rituals reinforce flow and renewal. Incorporate intentional practices—reflective visualizations, mindful journaling, or purposeful movement—so that the act of letting go becomes embodied, seamless, and fully aligned with your highest intentions.

Releasing old anchors is an ongoing practice that cultivates freedom, clarity, and emotional resilience. Each intentional step— no matter how small—reinforces your ability to move through life with openness, lightness, and conscious presence.

Key Affirmation:
I release what no longer serves me. I embrace clarity, flow, and the freedom to thrive.

⚙ PRACTICAL STEPS TO:
Release Old Baggage and Create Space

- **Identify What You Carry Daily** – Take a few moments each morning to notice any emotional or energetic weight. Acknowledge thoughts, tensions, or recurring patterns without judgment.

- **Pause and Breathe Into Release** – When old stories, resentment, or stress arise, inhale deeply, exhale slowly, and visualize letting go with each breath.

- **Ask:** *"What am I ready to release today?"* – Tune into feelings, attachments, or expectations holding you back. Reflect on what no longer serves your growth or well-being.

- **Journal Reflections and Take One Releasing Action –** Write down insights or emotions that surface. Choose a small, intentional act—like forgiving, decluttering, or expressing gratitude—to reinforce your release.

- **Notice Patterns and Celebrate Liberation –** Track repeated emotional or energetic themes over time. Recognize moments of lightness, celebrate progress, and allow letting go to become a conscious, embodied practice.

⛰ AWARENESS CHECKPOINTS

Check in with yourself throughout the day to notice where release is needed.

- Observe moments when old stories, resentment, or frustration arise—note how they show up physically, emotionally, or mentally.

- Identify repetitive triggers or situations that keep you anchored in past pain.

- Ask: ***"What am I holding onto that no longer serves me?"*** and notice your initial reactions.

- Track shifts in your energy after practicing letting go, noticing increased clarity, lightness, or openness.

🎯 INTENTIONS

By the end of Flight 7, you will:

- Identify emotional or energetic burdens you are holding onto.

- Observe situations where old stories, resentment, or expectations influence your reactions.

- Develop a daily practice to consciously release what no longer serves you.

- Approach your inner self with curiosity and compassion as you let go.

- Notice subtle cues in your body, mind, and emotions signaling stuck energy.

- Pause before reacting to triggers, allowing space for mindful release.

- Commit to small, consistent rituals that support energetic and emotional clearing.

- Recognize recurring patterns to understand what needs release.

- Strengthen trust in your capacity to create space for healing and renewal.

🧰 TOOLS & TECHNIQUES

Six key practices to support release, cultivate lightness, and create energetic space for growth.

✦ Forgiveness Ritual for Release ✦

Release resentment and reclaim peace through intentional self-compassion.

- Find a quiet, comfortable space and place one hand over your heart. Slowly say: ***"I forgive everyone who has ever hurt or harmed me. I offer them grace, peace, and understanding."***

- Inhale deeply, asking forgiveness for anything you may have done to cause harm, knowingly or unknowingly. As you inhale, welcome compassion; as you exhale, release guilt and regret.

- Place both hands over your heart and affirm:

  "I forgive myself.
  I accept grace and peace.
  I am free, happy, and healthy.
  I stand in my full power."

- Notice how your body softens as forgiveness expands, creating space for renewal and lightness.

✦ Forgiveness Through Writing ✦

Transform lingering emotions into clarity and freedom with pen and paper.

- Choose a quiet moment to write a forgiveness letter—to yourself, another person, or a challenging situation.

- Express your feelings honestly, acknowledging both the pain and your willingness to release it.

- Close with a statement of release, such as: ***"I let go. I choose peace and freedom."***

- When complete, symbolically release the letter by burning, shredding, or discarding it, imagining the heaviness dissolving.

✦ Forgiveness Through Tapping ✦

Free emotional energy through touch and spoken release.

- While seated comfortably, tap gently through the standard EFT (Emotional Freedom Technique) points.

- As you tap, repeat: ***"I acknowledge the pain and choose to forgive. I feel hurt, but I am ready to release this."***

- Continue tapping until you sense a softening, then close with: ***"I let go of blame and open my heart to healing."***

- Notice the calm or relief that follows as old energy shifts into spaciousness.

✦ Guided Release Visualization ✦

Use imagery to unburden your heart and invite lightness.

- Sit or lie down in a quiet space. Close your eyes and take slow, grounding breaths.

- Visualize yourself carrying a heavy suitcase filled with old pain, resentment, or outdated stories.

- See yourself setting it down and watching it dissolve, float away, or transform into golden light.

- Feel your body lighten as freedom and spaciousness flow in, replacing the old weight with clarity.

- Invite a soft wave of golden light to move through your entire body — from the crown of your head to the soles of your feet — cleansing, soothing, and renewing every cell.

- As this light flows, silently affirm: *"I release what no longer serves me. I am free to move forward with peace and purpose."*

- Take a few moments to notice the new sensations within — perhaps warmth, expansion, or stillness.

- Anchor this feeling of spaciousness by placing one hand over your heart and one over your abdomen, breathing gratitude into the present moment.

✦ Energetic Clearing Through Decluttering ✦

Create outer order to mirror and amplify inner freedom.

- Choose one small area—drawer, shelf, or closet—to clear. Move slowly and with intention.

- Keep only items that spark joy, usefulness, or alignment; release what feels heavy or unnecessary.

- As you donate, discard, or recycle items, notice the shift in your body and breath.

- Allow the outer clearing to reflect your inner release, opening new space for energy to flow.

✦ Daily Letting Go Meditation ✦

Anchor your practice of release with a simple, repeatable ritual.

- Find a comfortable seat, close your eyes, and breathe deeply until your body feels steady.

- Imagine a heavy weight dissolving into light with each exhale.

- Silently repeat:
  "I release what no longer serves me. I create space for healing and joy."

- Rest a few breaths, feeling lightness spread through your body.

- Open your eyes and carry that freedom into the rest of your day.

GUIDED PRACTICE:
Ritual of Release and Renewal

1. Find a quiet, comfortable space. Sit with your spine upright or lie down, allowing your body to relax.

2. Place one hand on your heart and the other on your belly. Take three slow, deep breaths—inhale through the nose, exhale through the mouth—settling into presence.

3. Bring to mind a burden: a painful memory, a resentment, or a limiting belief. Feel its weight without judgment.

4. Visualize it as a heavy object. Notice its shape, size, and texture.

5. With your breath, imagine placing this burden down before you. As you exhale, see it dissolve into light, carried away by wind, water, or fire. Repeat softly: *"I release you. I no longer carry what is not mine to hold."*

6. Pause in the empty space that remains. Feel the lightness in your body, the expansion in your chest, the freedom in your energy.

7. Invite renewal by silently affirming: *"I am free. I am open. I create space for healing, joy, and new beginnings."*

8. When you feel complete, open your eyes gently and journal any insights, sensations, or commitments that arose.

🧘 MEDITATION SCRIPT:

Guided Meditation for Releasing Emotional Triggers

Use a slow, calm voice when reading or recording this for yourself or others.

"Close your eyes. Bring your awareness to your breath.

Feel the natural rhythm of your inhale and exhale, flowing like waves on the shore.

Now, bring your attention to your heart. Place your left hand gently over it and then your right hand over your left.

Notice the sensations here—the warmth, the beat, the energy.

With each inhale, invite calmness, clarity, and compassion into your being.

With each exhale, release fear-based triggers—anger, judgment, doubt, or stress— letting them dissolve like mist in the morning sun.

*You can simply repeat the words **"let go"** in sync with your breath, inhaling and exhaling 9 times.*

Now, imagine a soft, radiant light glowing in the center of your heart.

*With every breath, this light expands, filling your chest, your entire body, and surrounding you in a cocoon of **love** and safety.*

Repeat silently to yourself:
*'I choose **love**. I release fear. I trust my inner strength. I let go of the past and choose to stay steeped in the present moment.'*

Take a few breaths here, letting the words sink into your heart and body.

By repeating this affirmation 3, 6, or 9 times, your subconscious program begins to change.

*When you feel complete, thank yourself for choosing **love** over fear.*

Take one final deep, grounding breath, smile gently, and open your eyes."

🛠 ADDITIONAL TOOLS

Daily practices to anchor liberation.

- **Morning Reset:** Hand on heart, ask:
  "What can I let go of today?"
  Start the day lighter.

- **Evening Note:** Write down one thing
  you released or handled differently.

- **Move It Out:** Stretch, shake, or take a
  quick walk to clear tension.

- **Pause for Freedom:** Take 1–2 minutes
  to breathe deeply, noticing what softens
  as you exhale.

- **Hydration Check:** As you drink water,
  picture it rinsing away stress and
  bringing clarity.

- **Grounding Outdoors:** Step onto grass, sand, or earth. Notice how steady it feels under you.

- **Light Bubble:** Imagine a calm space around you that keeps out what drains you and holds in what supports you.

🫥 REFLECTION PROMPTS

Use these prompts to deepen awareness and guide conscious action.

- What am I holding onto?

- How does it affect me physically, emotionally, and energetically?

- What will I release today?

- How will I create space for growth and healing?

- What small action can I take to practice letting go?

🛬 LANDING WISDOM:
Releasing Fear, Returning to Love

Choosing **love** over fear is the turning point of your healing journey. Each moment you pause and soften opens the door to deeper peace within yourself, creating space.

Fear may rise, but it no longer has to rule you. With awareness, you can meet it gently, release its grip, and choose again—this time in alignment with **love** and kindness.

Living from **love** restores your clarity, strengthens your relationships, and nurtures your body's natural ability to heal.

You are not defined by fear, you are carried by **love**, and **love** is your truest compass.

RECAP OF YOUR JOURNEY

Congratulations—you've completed Flight 7 of your healing journey. Your engines are lightened by release; your horizon is wide open for renewal.

Keep your navigation tuned to your heart, and remember:

Release the past, reclaim your light, rise with ease—*Flight 7 clears the skies for what's next.*

📝 AFFIRMATIONS FOR FLIGHT 7:

Freedom Through Release

Use these positive statements daily to nurture release, freedom, and renewal.

- I gently release what no longer serves my highest good.

- I trust the process of life and surrender with grace.

- Each breath I take frees me from old patterns and opens space for new beginnings.

- I let go of attachments and welcome peace into my heart.

- I forgive myself and others, creating space for healing and **love**.

- I choose freedom over fear and trust the path unfolding before me.

- I release control and allow life to move through me with ease.

- I let go of the past and step fully into the present moment.

- Every release lightens my spirit and aligns me with joy and renewal.

COMPANION WORKSHEET

COMPANION WORKSHEET

✈ Chapter 8:
HEALING THROUGH BELIEF & IMAGINATION

Flight 8 – Activating Your New Reality

🔑 KEY QUESTION / Allaine's Insight

What beliefs do I currently hold that support or limit my healing?

✈ SESSION OVERVIEW

Your beliefs are the code guiding your healing journey. This chapter teaches you how to harness the transformative power of affirmations, visualization, and conscious imagination to rewrite limiting beliefs and manifest your desired reality.

Engaging your mind's healing intelligence daily builds a resilient, empowered foundation for lifelong wellbeing. You'll practice imagining your highest potential and anchoring it through sensory-rich visualization, creating a blueprint for transformation. Daily engagement strengthens the subconscious mind, aligning your energy with your intentions.

KEY TERMS PREVIEW

Before takeoff, familiarize yourself with this essential terminology so you can integrate each practice effectively throughout Flight 8.

- **Scripting –** Writing your future self's experiences in present tense to reprogram the subconscious for success, gratitude, and empowerment.

- **Placebo Effect –** The mind's power to influence the body and outcomes through expectation, belief, and mental rehearsal.

- **Sensory Anchoring –** Engaging sight, sound, touch, taste, and smell to reinforce new beliefs and create embodied experiences of desired outcomes.

- **Liberation Practices –** Simple, repeatable actions that help you let go of stress, fear, or heaviness day by day.

- **Pattern Interruption –** Small, intentional shifts in behavior or thought that break old habits and open space for new ones.

- **Embodied Belief Integration –** Using posture, movement, or simple actions to make new beliefs feel real in your body and mind.

💡 CORE CONCEPTS

Before takeoff, here are the vital essentials:

- Beliefs shape biology, behavior, and overall life experience.

- Conscious visualization reprograms limiting beliefs and aligns energy to desired outcomes.

- Affirmations and scripting strengthen neuroplasticity and create lasting subconscious change.

- Interrupting limiting patterns with empowering ones, shifts energy.

- Daily practices integrate mind, body, and spirit, for clarity and alignment.

📅 DETAILED ITINERARY

Let's explore the chapter's key ideas.

Our minds shape experiences and influence the body's healing. Beliefs act like software guiding the nervous system, immune responses, and cellular function. Visualization trains brain and body, showing that imagining yourself whole and healthy triggers real change—the placebo effect in action.

Shifting from limiting beliefs like "I am stuck" to affirmations such as ***"I am worthy of vibrant health."*** opens new possibilities.

Engaging all senses strengthens the subconscious and energetic field. Healing is both mental and energetic; consistent practice moves you from resistance to openness, vitality, and alignment with your highest self.

🔍 DEEP DIVE: Shifting Perceptions

Let's look closer at the core insight.

Recognizing Limiting Thoughts

Our minds often run on autopilot, repeating assumptions and ideas we've accepted as truths. Notice thoughts that trigger stress, doubt, or self-criticism. By identifying these patterns, you can pause before they shape your emotions or actions.

Awareness is the first step in shifting from automatic reactions to intentional responses.

Replacing with Empowering Alternatives

Once limiting thoughts are recognized, replace them with supportive statements or visions. Small, consistent mental shifts compound over time, rewiring neural pathways and reinforcing confidence, clarity, and possibility.

Anchoring New Perceptions in Daily Life

Integration is key—practice your new perspectives in real situations. Notice how your reactions, decisions, and energy change when you operate from empowering mindsets. Journaling, reflection, and micro-pauses throughout the day strengthen these new pathways. The more consistently you anchor these perceptions, the more naturally your reality begins to align with them.

Shifting your perceptions helps you move from limits to clarity and possibility. Consistently choosing new perspectives creates positive change in your mind and life.

Key Affirmation:
I notice my thoughts, choose empowering perspectives, and align my mind with my highest potential.

⚙️ PRACTICAL STEPS TO:
Turn On the Placebo Effect

- **Affirm With Feeling** – Speak your chosen affirmations slowly and with belief. Fully feel the emotion behind each statement.
  Example:
  "I am whole, healthy, and vibrant."

- **Visualize in Detail** – Engage all your senses to imagine yourself fully healed, joyful, and free. See it, hear it, feel it, and embody it as if it's real now.

- **Create a Healing Script** – Write a detailed narrative of your future self living your healthiest life in present tense. Immerse your subconscious in this reality.

- **Repeat Consistently** – Practice daily, even for a few minutes. Repetition compounds over time, reinforcing your mind-body connection.

- **Integrate Physical and Energetic Actions** – Pair visualization with gentle movement, breathwork, or energy practices to deepen the experience and anchor healing.

⚖️ AWARENESS CHECKPOINTS

Take out your journal and put pen to paper.

- Notice recurring thoughts or beliefs that feel limiting or disempowering.

- Observe emotional reactions tied to old patterns or self-judgments.

- Pay attention to how your body responds to empowering versus limiting thoughts.

- Tune into moments when imagination or visualization shifts your energy or perspective.

- Track subtle changes in confidence, clarity, or motivation after daily affirmations and belief work.

🎯 INTENTIONS

By the end of Flight 8, you will:

- Identify limiting or disempowering beliefs that influence your healing journey.

- Take introspective moments to notice how thoughts shape emotions and energy.

- Develop a daily affirmation and visualization practice to reinforce empowerment.

- Embrace curiosity and openness as you explore new possibilities for growth.

- Cultivate awareness of subtle shifts in confidence, clarity, and motivation.

- Practice pausing to consciously replace old patterns with empowering alternatives.

- Commit to small, consistent daily exercises that strengthen belief in your potential.

- Notice patterns in emotional and energetic responses to thoughts and imagination.

- Strengthen trust in your mind's creative power and inner guidance.

💼 TOOLS & TECHNIQUES

Here are six practical exercises to strengthen your awareness, rewire limiting patterns, and support your mental, emotional, and physical well-being.

✦ Heart-Centered Visualization ✦
Engage your inner guidance and imagine your healed self fully.

- Find a quiet space, sit comfortably, spine upright yet relaxed.

- Before you begin heart centered visualization, you may wish to cover your eyes so you do not get distracted.

- Close your eyes and take 5 slow, deep breaths, settling into stillness.

- Visualize yourself fully healed, vibrant, and confident, engaging all your senses.

- Sense emotions, energy, and physical sensations as if this reality is happening now.

- Your deep understanding of feeling the exact desired outcome you wish for, *in the present moment*, allows you to connect with your new reality.

- Record insights or feelings in your journal after the practice.

- Before you begin heart centered visualization, you may wish to cover your eyes, so you do not get distracted.

✦ Daily Affirmation Practice ✦

Check in with your body to notice subtle signals and start your day grounded.

- Choose 1–2 affirmations that resonate deeply, such as:
  "I am fully healthy and strong."

- Repeat slowly, out loud or silently, feeling each word in your body.

- Notice subtle shifts in thought, energy, or emotion as you recite.

- Reflect briefly afterward in your journal to track breakthroughs and patterns.

✦ Future Self Scripting ✦

Write your desired reality into existence.

- Each morning or evening, write as if you're healed, ideal self is living fully.

- Include feelings, accomplishments, relationships, and wellbeing in present tense.

- Read your script aloud, immerse yourself in the emotions, and visualize embodying it.

- Revise and expand daily to reinforce belief and imagination pathways.

✨ **Reflective Healing Walks** ✨

Combine movement with conscious imagination, affirmation, and sensory awareness.

- Mindfully walk in nature, repeating chosen affirmations or focusing on intentions, letting each step connect you to your inner guidance.

- Engage your senses, notice the colors, patterns, textures, sounds, smells, and subtle energy shifts around and within you, allowing the environment to amplify your awareness.

- Observe thoughts, insights, or creative ideas that arise naturally, noticing how your body, breath, and emotions respond in real time.

✦ Sensory Immersion Practice ✦

Bring your visualizations and affirmations to life by fully engaging your senses and body.

- When visualizing, notice textures, smells, sounds, and even tastes associated with your desired reality, allowing each detail to feel vivid and present.

- Imagine yourself moving, speaking, or interacting in this healed state, observing posture, gestures, and energy as if it is happening right now.

- Anchor these impressions with a few slow breaths or gentle movements, deepening the belief and embodiment of your healed self.

✦ Symbolic Release Ritual ✦

Turn limiting beliefs into tangible energy you can let go of.

- Write down a belief or story you want to release, noticing how it feels in your body and mind as you put it on paper.

- Safely burn, tear, or bury it while saying: **"I release this; I make space for my healed, authentic self."**

- Feel the shift in your energy as tension, heaviness, or resistance lifts, creating space for clarity, peace, and empowerment.

- Express gratitude for the release, acknowledging the strength it took to let go!

- Close the ritual by placing both hands over your heart and repeating:

  "I am free.
  I am whole.
  I am ready for what's next."

- Spend a few quiet moments in stillness, noticing the spaciousness and calm that follow.

📖 GUIDED PRACTICE:
Embody Your Healed Self

1. Find a quiet, comfortable space where you can sit or lie undisturbed.

2. Close your eyes and take three slow, grounding breaths, feeling your body settle.

3. Recall one limiting belief or story you want to shift.

4. Reframe it with an empowering *"Why"* question affirmation, such as:
   "Why am I naturally confident and strong?" or
   "Why am I fully aligned with my healthiest, happiest self?"

5. Visualize this affirmation as radiant, golden light spreading through your body, mind, and energy field.

6. Engage your senses: feel movement, hear sounds, notice textures, and sense the emotions of your healed self. Let the vision feel real and present.

7. Imagine yourself living your desired reality for a full day—acting, speaking, and moving as your empowered self.

8. Repeat the affirmation slowly three times, breathing deeply and noticing shifts in sensation, emotion, or energy.

9. Open your eyes and record any insights or feelings in your journal.

🧘 MEDITATION SCRIPT:

Embodying Your Empowered Self

Use a slow, calm voice when reading or recording this for yourself or others.

"Close your eyes. Bring your attention to your heart.

Feel the gentle rise and fall of your chest and your lower belly.

Imagine an extra set of nostrils in your chest and your belly button.

Watch the expansion of your chest and abdomen several times until you feel calm, open, and present.

Visualize a warm, golden light above you, like the sun or moonlight, shining down.

With each inhale, breathe in this healing, vibrant energy.

With each exhale, release limiting beliefs, doubts, or fears—letting go of what no longer serves you.

Now, ask yourself:

'What empowered vision of myself can I embody today?'

Take time to imagine yourself fully healed, vibrant, and confident.

Engage your senses—see, hear, and feel yourself living this reality.

Trust the images, sensations, and insights that arise.

Let them guide you naturally.

When ready, thank yourself for this practice, take one or two deep, grounding breaths, and slowly open your eyes.

Carry this renewed energy into your day or night.

Perhaps you feel drawn to journal or record any messages that presented themselves during this mediation.

Be sure to have your journal and pen handy."

🛠️ ADDITIONAL TOOLS

Key practices to strengthen your beliefs, imagination, and healing energy.

- **Morning Mindset Alignment:** Set one intention for your day that reflects your highest self.

- **Evening Reflection & Release:** Write down a limiting thought you noticed and consciously let it go.

- **Creative Visualization:** Spend 2–3 minutes vividly imagining yourself achieving a goal or feeling fully healed.

- **Affirmation Walks:** Repeat your chosen affirmation while moving, noticing how your body responds.

- **Energy Checkpoints:** Pause midday to sense where your energy feels blocked or inspired and adjust focus.

- **Senses Reboot:** Engage all five senses intentionally—smell, touch, sight, sound, taste—to ground yourself in the present.

- **Imagination Journaling:** Record new ideas, insights, or mental images that support your growth.

- **Empowered Pause:** Before responding to stress, visualize a protective bubble of light and respond from clarity.

🫣 REFLECTION PROMPTS

Use these prompts to explore your beliefs, notice patterns, and envision your healed, empowered self.

- What beliefs support or limit my healing?

- How does imagination change my experience of these beliefs?

- Which feelings or sensory details make my affirmations feel real?

- What does my scripted future-self look and feel like?

- What is one small step I can take today to align beliefs with my healing vision?

🛬 LANDING WISDOM:
Harnessing Your Inner Vision

Your beliefs and imagination shape your reality.

Each intentional thought and visualization strengthen your ability to heal and manifest positive change.

This journey is ongoing—cultivating awareness, rewiring old patterns, and envisioning the life you desire. Consistent practice aligns your mind, body, and energy, creating lasting transformation.

Your inner vision is your guide. Trust it, nurture it, and let it illuminate the path to your highest potential.

RECAP OF YOUR JOURNEY

Congratulations — you've completed Flight 8 of your healing journey. Your mind, heart, and imagination are now aligned, guiding your reality with intention.

Keep your focus tuned to your inner vision, and remember:

Thoughts aligned, beliefs empowered, imagination activated — *this flight sets the course for creating the life you desire.*

📝 AFFIRMATIONS FOR FLIGHT 8:
Manifesting Your Best Self

Use these positive statements daily to nurture awareness, trust, and healing.

- I trust my mind's power to shape my reality and support my healing.

- I embrace empowering beliefs that guide me toward vibrant health and joy.

- My imagination creates positive, tangible changes in my life and body.

- I align my thoughts, feelings, and actions with my highest well-being.

- I see myself fully healed, confident, and thriving in every moment.

- My beliefs and intentions naturally attract balance, abundance, and vitality.

- I release limiting thoughts and replace them with empowering possibilities.

- I nurture my inner healer through consistent practice and awareness.

- Every affirmation strengthens my alignment with health, clarity, and joy.

✈ Chapter 9:
HEAL THYSELF FIRST

Flight 9 – Embodying Your Healing to Lead Others

🔑 KEY QUESTION / Allaine's Insight

Are you a healer in a wounded body?

✈ SESSION OVERVIEW

Over four decades of guiding beautiful souls, I've witnessed a profound truth: most of us did not arrive on this path by accident. We were called here—through pain, illness, unexplainable challenges, or a quiet inner knowing that life is more than survival and fight-or-flight.

This chapter is a sacred invitation to become your own healer first. As you integrate these practices daily, powerful shifts arise from within, building clarity, strength, and inner peace.

For those called to share this work professionally, an opportunity for certification and CEUs equips you to lead with authenticity and heart.

KEY TERMS PREVIEW

Keep these essentials in mind to make the most of Flight 9:

- **Inner Resonance** —Attune deeply to the subtle signals of your body, mind, and heart. Notice sensations, shifts in emotion, and intuitive nudges, allowing these inner messages to guide your decisions, actions, and interactions with clarity, authenticity, and grounded presence.

- **Energetic Alignment** – Bringing your internal energy, intentions, beliefs, and actions into harmony, fostering a sense of flow, mental clarity, emotional balance, and vibrant vitality throughout your being.

- **Healing Frequency** – The vibrational quality of your body and energy; a consistent state of balance enhances self-healing and supports others.

- **Self-Leadership** – Leading yourself first through awareness, alignment, and intentional action; the prerequisite for guiding or supporting others effectively.

- **Compassionate Presence** – Engaging with yourself and others from a state of understanding, empathy, and non-judgment.

- **Embodied Wisdom** – Knowledge gained from integrated body-mind-spirit awareness; guides decisions, interactions, and leadership from authenticity.

CORE CONCEPTS

Before takeoff, here are the vital essentials:

- Healing yourself first creates the foundation for guiding and supporting others authentically.

- Where attention goes, energy follows; calm and alignment build trust.

- Boundaries protect your energy and support sustainable giving.

- Consistent daily practices of awareness, reflection, and ritual embed healing into your life and work.

- Your aligned body, mind, and spirit naturally inspire, guide, and positively influence those around you.

▦ DETAILED ITINERARY

Let's explore the chapter's key ideas.

For many, healing begins with a wound—not to punish, but to reveal a deeper invitation. This sparks willingness to step into the role of healer, guide, or caretaker.

Authentic journeys unfold as you reclaim power—releasing limiting stories and embracing your true potential.

By integrating body wisdom, emotional flow, energy shielding, choosing **love** over fear, and belief work, you align with your limitless self. This alignment creates a vibrational match for health, wholeness, and purpose, inviting you to open your heart and mind to your unique vision—the new you.

🔍 DEEP DIVE: Healing Awareness

Let's look closer at the core insight.

The **Listening to Subtle Signals -** Your body communicates before illness, pain, or fatigue appears. Paying attention to minor shifts—like tension, heaviness, or rapid breath—helps you respond before imbalance escalates. These early whispers guide choices that keep energy flowing and prevent overwhelm.

Presence Over Reaction - Healing Awareness is about observing without judgment. Like a pilot adjusting to subtle wind changes, you can respond calmly rather than reacting from fear or stress. This transforms survival patterns into intentional, conscious action, fostering clarity, resilience, and balance.

Consistent Practice Builds Resilience

Daily check-ins, journaling, and mindful pauses strengthen body-mind connection. Small, consistent actions—breathwork, energy resets, or reflection—retrain the nervous system and support lasting physical, emotional, and energetic alignment. Over time, these habits cultivate wholeness, presence, and the capacity to lead from healing.

By paying close attention and being present, you build a strong and steady wholeness. Daily practice makes your body, mind, and energy stronger, helping you heal and lead with clarity and compassion.

Key Affirmation:

I listen, respond, and align with my body's wisdom, embodying healing and wholeness.

⚙ PRACTICAL STEPS TO:
Facilitate Daily Healing

- **Check-In Pause** – Three times daily, ask: *"What is my body saying? - My heart feeling? - My mind thinking?"* Notice subtle shifts without judgment.

- **Sensory Scan** – Tune into one thing you can see, hear, feel, smell, and taste to anchor yourself in the present moment.

- **Early Signal Journal** – Record early signs of imbalance and what helps shift them; observe patterns over time.

- **Energy Baseline** – Each morning, rate your energy 1–10 and note quality; use this as a guide for mid-day recalibration.

- **Micro-Alignment** – When feeling "off," take 60 seconds to adjust: deep breath, posture correction, sip of water, or repeat a grounding mantra such as *"I return to my center."*

- **Evening Integration** – Before bed, reflect on moments of presence and awareness, noting successes and insights to reinforce daily practice.

- **Consistent Practice & Repetition** – Cultivate positive thoughts and feelings daily, knowing that repetition rewires the mind, strengthens resilience, and deepens lasting transformation.

🏛️ AWARENESS CHECKPOINTS

Pause, breathe, and tune into your body, mind, and heart.

- Am I listening to my body and heart before acting or reacting?

- Where have I given away my healing power or ignored my own needs?

- Which external pressures have influenced my sense of balance and wellness?

- How can I trust my body's guidance and inner wisdom more fully?

- What small, intentional actions can I take today to honor my healing and presence?

◎ INTENTIONS

By the end of Flight 9, you will:

- Identify and reflect on origins of disharmony in your life, exploring how these roots have shaped your physical, emotional, and energetic wellbeing.

- Observe the moments when you experience energetic depletion or blocks, becoming aware of how they limit your natural flow, creativity, and vitality.

- Use journaling, meditation, tapping, and grounding to clear blocks.

- Weave masterclass teachings into daily rituals embodying healing and presence.

- Cultivate authentic leadership through consistent, aligned actions.

- Teach and share from a place of healing rather than from unprocessed wounds, centering your guidance in vulnerability, compassion, and truth.

- Build a sustainable self-healing practice supporting personal and professional growth.

- Recognize recurring patterns in your relationships, work, or inner dialogue, and use these insights as opportunities for transformation and liberation.

🧰 TOOLS & TECHNIQUES

Here are six practical exercises to deepen your healing, release limiting patterns, and support your mental, emotional, and physical renewal.

❋ Heart-Centered Alignment ❋

Reconnect with your inner healer and cultivate grounded presence.

- Find a quiet, comfortable space where you won't be disturbed. Sit with your spine upright yet relaxed.

- Place your left hand over your heart and your right hand gently on top.

- Close your eyes and take 5 slow, deep breaths.

- Focus on your heartbeat and silently ask:

  "What does my body most need from me today?"

- Listen without judgment, allowing insights, sensations, or images to arise.

- Record reflections in your journal to honor the messages received.

✦ Somatic Presence Ritual ✦

Deepen your connection to your body and awaken your inner healer.

- Start your day by standing or sitting comfortably, closing your eyes, and taking three slow, intentional breaths.

- Scan your body for tension, energy, or subtle sensations.

- Gently place your hands over any area that calls for attention, silently sending warmth, presence, and compassion.

- Notice any shifts or releases, honoring them without judgment.

- Set an intention for your day, carrying awareness and balance forward.

✦ Spinal Breath Alignment ✦

Awaken your body's central channel and restore flow.

- Sit tall, sensing the natural curve of your spine from tailbone to crown.

- Inhale gently, imagining breath rising upward along your spine.

- Pause at the crown, sensing spaciousness and clarity.

- Exhale slowly, guiding the breath downward, releasing tension into the earth.

- Continue for several cycles, attuning to balance between rooted stability and expanded awareness.

✦ Mirror Work – Embodying Your Wholeness ✦

Cultivate self-compassion and acknowledge your healing journey.

- Stand before a mirror in a quiet space. Let shoulders relax and take a slow, deep breath.

- Look into your own eyes, noticing any emotion without judgment. Speak a kind affirmation, such as:

  "I am whole." or **"I honor my growth."**

- If resistance arises, observe it as a signal to nurture yourself gently.

- Stay 1–3 minutes, letting your words settle into your heart.

- Notice how your body responds — a warmth in the chest, a tear, or a softening of your breath — all signs of release and integration.

- Close the practice by smiling at yourself, affirming:

"I see you.
I love you.
I am proud of how far you've come."

- Journal any insights, emotions, or sensations that arose, allowing your reflections to anchor your sense of inner wholeness.

✦ Sacred Dialogue with Self ✦

Transform journaling into a practice of communion with your inner wisdom.

- Instead of recounting your day, write a conversation between your present self and your inner guide, body, or heart.

- Write as if you are speaking directly with your inner guide, heart, or body, exploring thoughts, doubts, and emotions.

- Allow questions, doubts, and emotions to flow—then listen for answers that arise from within.

- Close by highlighting one truth or insight that feels like a compass point for your journey forward.

✦ Evening Healing Practice ✦

Close the day with intention, gratitude, and restoration.

- Before sleep, note three things you are grateful for—about yourself, your body, or your life—feeling each one in your body.

- Set one clear, positive intention for tomorrow, visualizing it with detail, emotion, and presence.

- Close with a few deep breaths, sensing your body, mind, and spirit aligned and at ease.

- This ritual restores energy, supports healing, and alignment.

GUIDED PRACTICE:
Embodying Wholeness

1. Find a sacred, quiet space that feels nourishing to your soul. Sit upright or lie down, allowing your body to be fully supported.

2. Place your left hand over your heart and the right hand over your lower belly, uniting your breath with the rhythm of life within you.

3. Close your eyes and take three long, intentional breaths. With each inhale, receive positive energy. With each exhale, release all that no longer belongs to you.

4. Bring to mind an area of your life or body where you've felt separate, wounded, or incomplete. Simply witness it without judgment, as a compassionate observer.

5. Now, gently whisper:
   "I am whole. I am complete. I am healed."

   Allow these words to vibrate through every cell, every organ, every part of your being.

6. Visualize a radiant light—golden, expansive, infinite—flowing from your heart outward, filling the space within and around you. Notice how it dissolves the illusion of separation and restores you to your natural state of wholeness.

7. Rest in this presence for several breaths. Feel the union of body, mind, and spirit as one seamless flow of life.

8. When you're ready, slowly open your eyes. Write down one insight, one truth, or one affirmation you want to carry forward as you embody your healing in everyday life.

🧘 MEDITATION SCRIPT:

Guided Meditation for Embodying Your Healing

Use a steady, gentle voice when reading or recording this for yourself or others.

"Close your eyes. Feel the earth beneath you, steady and unshakable.

Sense the weight of your body resting fully into this moment, nothing to prove, nothing to fix.

Bring your left hand over your heart and your right hand over your left.

Feel its rhythm, the eternal drum of life within you. Repeat silently to yourself:
'I am grateful. I am alive. I am whole. I am here.'

Now, imagine a luminous thread of light rising from your heart into the vastness above you.

See it stretch into the infinite sky, connecting you with the source of all creation—pure **love**, pure wisdom, pure healing.

With each inhale, draw in this radiant light, filling every cell, every organ, every hidden corner of your being.

With each exhale, release what no longer serves—old stories, wounds, judgments, and fears—letting them dissolve into the horizon.

Feel yourself expanding—your body, your energy, your spirit—becoming spacious, free, and deeply at peace. Now, vision yourself standing in front of a mirror of light.

Look deeply. See not just your reflection, but your healed self, the version of you who has walked through fire, embraced the lessons, and now radiates wisdom and compassion.

Ask this healed self:
'How will you guide me forward?
How will you lead?'

Wait. Listen. Trust. Whatever arises is your truth.

When you are ready, bring your awareness back to your heart. Bow inward with gratitude—for the journey, for your resilience, for the light you now carry.

Take one deep, nourishing breath, and when you feel complete, slowly open your eyes—returning as both healer and healed, ready to live, lead, and **love**."

🛠️ ADDITIONAL TOOLS

Key practices to carry-on into each day.

- **Protective Visualization**: Envision a radiant bubble of light around you before entering challenging spaces.

- **Nature Reset**: Spend 10 minutes outside daily, letting the earth re-balance your body, mind, and spirit.

- **Hydration Ritual**: Hold your water or nourishing drink with intention, offering a silent blessing before each sip.

- **Heart Check-In**: Pause mid-day, place a hand over your heart, and ask, *"What is most alive in me right now?"*

- **Evening Reflection**: Write down one subtle message your body or spirit offered you that day.

- **Release Stretch**: Gentle, mindful movements to invite softness and dissolve stored tension before bed.

- **Light Invocation**: Imagine calling in soft golden light as you rest, allowing it to cleanse and restore your inner world.

🧖 REFLECTION PROMPTS

Use these prompts to embody your own healing and lead with greater clarity.

- Where do I most often feel imbalance? *What is it trying to tell me?*

- What are earliest signals before physical or emotional drain?

- How can I honor these signals sooner?

- Which daily ritual keeps me grounded and aligned?

- How will my healing journey inspire guiding others?

🛬 LANDING WISDOM:
Embodying Your Healing

Your healing is not separate from your leadership—it begins in your own body. Each choice to rest, nourish, and honor your needs becomes an act of alignment with **love** over fear.

This path is not about perfection, but devotion—listening deeply, trusting the signals within, and responding with compassion. When you embody healing, you shine as a living example. Your presence alone becomes medicine for others, reminding them that wholeness is possible.

Your body is not a barrier to leadership, it is the very vessel that carries your wisdom into the world.

🗒️ RECAP OF YOUR JOURNEY

Congratulations — you've completed Flight 9 and landed with greater clarity, resilience, and trust in your healing path.

Your inner compass is awakened, your body's wisdom reclaimed, and your spirit aligned for the road ahead.

Remember: healing is not a destination but a lifelong flight—each choice, each practice, each moment of presence keeps you soaring toward wholeness.

You are ready to embody your healing and guide others by living as the fullest expression of yourself.

✒️ AFFIRMATIONS FOR FLIGHT 9:
Embodying Your Healing to Lead Others

Use these positive statements daily to embody wholeness, radiance, and authentic leadership.

- I embody my healing and shine it into the world with grace.

- My presence uplifts, inspires, and creates space for others to heal.

- I lead by example, rooted in **love**, truth, and compassion.

- Every breath strengthens my alignment with purpose and service.

- I trust the wisdom of my journey and share it with humility.

- My wholeness is a gift I offer to my community and beyond.

- I honor my body, mind, and spirit as sacred instruments of light.

- **Love** flows through me, guiding my words, actions, and leadership.

- I am a beacon of healing, resilience, and radiant authenticity.

APPENDIX

☀ *MEDITATION: TO KNOW THYSELF* ☀

Meditation is not about forcing the mind to be silent, nor is it about escaping the world.

Meditation is about turning inward to meet yourself fully.

It is a sacred act of self-knowledge, of peeling back the layers of thought, memory, and story, until only the essence of who you are remains.

When you meditate, you are not trying to become something else—calmer, wiser, more spiritual. *You are simply returning to yourself.*

You are listening to your own breath, watching the movement of your own mind, feeling the rhythm of your own heart.

In doing so, you remember: everything you need is already within you.

To meditate is to know thyself. It is the courage to sit in stillness and discover what lies beneath the noise.

It is allowing the truth of your being to reveal itself. This truth may come softly, like a whisper, or powerfully, like a wave. Either way, it is always there, waiting.

A Gentle Way to Begin

1. **Sit quietly.** Choose a space where you feel safe and supported. Sit comfortably with your spine tall, shoulders soft, and hands resting on your lap or heart.

2. **Close your eyes and breathe.** Let the breath flow naturally, as if it is breathing you. With each inhale, invite yourself home. With each exhale, release what is not you.

3. **Witness yourself.** Instead of chasing thoughts away, simply notice them. Notice feelings, sensations, memories, or silence. All are part of you. Welcome them with kindness.

4. **Rest in awareness.** Beyond the thoughts and emotions, there is a quiet watcher — the awareness that notices everything. Rest there. This awareness is who you truly are.

5. **Return gently.** When you feel complete, take a few deeper breaths. Open your eyes slowly. Carry this self-connection with you into your day.

✦ An Invitation

Do not worry about "doing it right." There is no wrong way to meet yourself.

Meditation is not a test. It is a relationship — a loving reunion with your own soul.

Even a few minutes each day creates a doorway back to your inner wisdom.

The more you enter, the more familiar it becomes, and the easier it is to live from that place of truth.

⁕ Final Reflection on Meditation

Meditation is the journey inward. It is the path of knowing thyself, of remembering that you are whole, radiant, and complete.

When you sit in silence, you are not trying to become more.

You are uncovering what has always been—
your true self.

TESLA 3-6-9 METHOD

The 3-6-9 Method is a simple daily ritual of writing a clear intention 3 times in the morning, 6 times at midday, and 9 times in the evening.

The repetition, clarity, emotion and simple ritual create focused attention, stronger intention, and practical momentum toward what you want.

Here is everything you need—background, why it works, exact step-by-step instructions, ready templates, variations, a 21-day plan, troubleshooting, and ethical notes.

Quick Note on Origins

People often link this practice to Nikola Tesla because he famously said the numbers 3, 6 and 9 were important. That historical link is interesting but not necessary.

What matters is how the practice functions as a modern ritual for attention and action.

Treat Tesla as inspiration, not scientific proof.

Why This Method Can Feel Powerful

- **Focus:** Repeating a clear statement keeps your mind pointed at one outcome instead of scattered.

- **Memory encoding:** Writing repeatedly helps your brain store and recall the intention more strongly.

- **Emotional tagging:** When you write with feeling, your brain connects emotion to the goal. Emotion motivates action.

- **Implementation intention:** The ritual trains you to notice opportunities and take small steps that move you toward the goal.

- **Habits and momentum:** A short, repeated ritual is easy to keep, and small repeated actions compound into progress.

This powerful method combines attention, feeling, memory and habit into a compact daily practice.

Core Principles to Use Every Time

1. **Be specific.** "I have more peace" is fine. "I make $10,000 this month" is fine. Vague like "better things" is weaker.

2. **Present tense.** Write as if it's already happening: *"I am..., I have..., I feel..."*

3. **Include feeling or outcome.** Add one emotion or concrete result: "calm, confident, 3 new clients"

4. **Short and repeatable.** One sentence you can quickly write 3, 6 and 9 times.

Pair with small action. After writing, decide on one tiny step you will take toward it.

✱ Step-by-Step Daily 3-6-9 Ritual

Before You Start: Pick your intention for the day or for a short period (week, month).

Keep a dedicated journal or notebook.

1. **Set up** — Find a quiet two minutes. Sit comfortably. Take three slow grounding breaths. With each inhale, invite calm and clarity; with each exhale, release any tension or distraction.

2. **Form your statement** — Make a single sentence using the rules above: specific, present tense, emotional if possible.

   Example: *"I am attracting three new ideal clients this month and I feel confident and organized."*

3. **Write 3 times (morning)** — Within the first hour of waking, write your sentence

4. **3 times**, slowly, by hand if possible. Pause briefly after each line and feel it.

5. **Write 6 times (midday)** — Around noon or the middle of your workday, write it **6 times**. Read each line out loud if you can.

6. **Write 9 times (evening)** — Before bed, write it **9 times**, again slowly. Conclude with one line of gratitude: "Thank you for this unfolding."

7. **Take one action** — After each session decide on one tiny action related to the intention and do it within 24 hours. Even a one-minute action counts.

8. **Reflection** — At the end of the week read your entries, note any ideas or opportunities that came up, and adjust the statement if needed.

Total practice time per day: about 5–12 minutes.

✦ Templates and Sample Statements

Use these patterns and adjust/customize them to your life.

Formats:

- I am [result], and I feel [feeling].

- I have [specific outcome] by [approximate timeframe].

- I am [quality] and this allows me to [action or outcome].

Examples:

- "I am attracting three ideal clients this month and I feel calm and confident."

- "I am in vibrant health, sleeping 7 hours, practicing gentle movement daily."

- "I am growing my email list to 1,000 people so I can serve more students."

✦ A Ready-to-Use Script You Can Use Today

Morning:
"I am attracting three ideal clients this month and I feel calm and confident." — write 3 times, pause, breathe.

Midday:
Same sentence — write 6 times, read out loud, say one small next step.

Evening:
Same sentence — write 9 times, add "Thank you," review one thing you did that moved it forward.

Variations and Ways to Deepen the Practice

- **Mirror work:** Say the sentence to yourself in the mirror while writing.

- **Voice recording:** Speak and save voice memos you can play later.

- **Visual anchor:** Add a small sketch, symbol or sticker next to each set of lines so your brain pairs the image with the intention.

- **Combine with breath:** Take three grounding breaths before each set, and end with a long exhale.

- **Movement:** Add a physical gesture after writing, like placing your hands over your heart or doing gentle stretches.

- **Sound healing:** After writing, hum or sing a small mantra to "settle" the intention in your body.

- **Alternate medium:** Write on paper one day, type in a dedicated app another day, speak another day — the variety can keep things fresh.

21-Day Micro Plan

- Days 1–7
  Choose one clear intention, follow full 3-6-9 daily ritual, track the one action each time.

- Days 8–14
  Review, refine the statement, increase your small actions, add mirror work or breath practice.

- Days 15–21
  Keep the ritual, focus on measurable steps and celebrate small wins. Journal insights weekly.

Measure progress by tracking: mood, ideas, concrete steps completed, small wins.

✦ Troubleshooting — Common Mistakes and Fixes

- **Vague intentions.** Fix: make it concrete and tangible.

- **Writing without feeling.** Fix: add an emotional word or imagine the scene for 20 seconds before writing.

- **Impatience.** Fix: remember this builds. attention and habits. Results may be subtle, showing up as new actions or fresh opportunities.

- **Using negatives.** Fix: don't write "I will not be anxious." Instead write "I am calm and confident."

✦ Ethical and Practical Notes

- Don't use this to try to control other people's free will or to harm anyone.

- Use it for personal growth, skill building, relationships that require mutual consent.

- If something is urgent or serious — health, legal, financial — pair intentions with competent professional action.

Short Scientific Note

There's no magical guarantee.

The 3-6-9 method's effectiveness most likely comes from psychological steps: clear goals, repeated practice, emotional focus, and inspired actions.

Those ingredients reliably change behavior. Treat the method like a short, elegant toolkit for attention and momentum.

EFT Tapping Technique: Healing with Your Fingertips

Emotional Freedom Technique or EFT, is a mind-body method that combines gentle tapping on specific points of the body with spoken words or affirmations.

It's sometimes called *psychological acupressure* because it borrows from Chinese medicine's meridian system but requires no needles.

Think of it as a reset button:
You acknowledge what you're feeling, calm the body's stress response, and then replace limiting thoughts with empowering ones.

Why EFT Works

- **Stress Reset:** Tapping sends calming signals to the brain (especially the amygdala), helping reduce fight-or-flight.

- **Acknowledgement + Acceptance:** Naming the feeling out loud reduces resistance and shame. "What we resist persists."

- **Rewiring:** Pairing old triggers with calm signals helps the brain form new responses.

- **Empowerment:** Repeating positive reframes while calm helps build new belief patterns.

✦ The Core EFT Sequence (Step-by-Step)

1. Choose your issue
Pick one clear issue at a time (stress, craving, fear, pain, etc.). Be specific: "I feel anxious before presenting at work," not just "I feel bad."

2. Rate your intensity
On a scale from 0–10, rate how strongly you feel it. This gives you a before-and-after measure.

3. The setup statement (karate chop point)
Tap on the *side of your hand* (the fleshy edge, below your pinky) and say three times:
"Even though I [describe the problem], I deeply and completely accept myself."
Example: "Even though I feel nervous about this meeting, I deeply and completely accept myself."

4. The tapping points

Using two fingers, gently tap each spot 5–7 times while saying a short reminder phrase (keeps you focused on the issue).

Here's the sequence (always top to bottom):

- **Eyebrow (EB):** inner edge of the eyebrow

- **Side of Eye (SE):** bone at the outer corner of the eye

- **Under Eye (UE):** bone under the eye

- **Under Nose (UN):** between nose and upper lip

- **Chin (CH):** crease below the bottom lip

- **Collarbone (CB):** just under the collarbone bone

- **Under Arm (UA):** side of body about 4 inches below armpit

- **Top of Head (TH):** crown of the head

5. Reminder phrase

While tapping each point, say a short version of your issue: "This nervous feeling" ... "So much pressure" ... "This fear in my chest."

6. Re-rate your intensity

After one or two rounds, pause. Rate your feeling again. Often it drops. Repeat as needed until it's down to 0–2.

7. Positive reframe (optional)

Once intensity lowers, add a new phrase as you tap: "I am calm now" ... "I choose to trust myself" ... "I am safe and grounded."

Sample EFT Script for Stress & Anxiety

This EFT sequence is designed for moments of stress and anxiety, when the mind feels scattered and the body carries tension.

The intention is to first acknowledge the stress honestly, so it no longer controls from the shadows, and then gently guide the nervous system into calm.

By naming the pressure and pairing it with soothing affirmations, the tapping helps shift the body from fight-or-flight into balance, allowing space for clarity, peace, and self-trust.

Step 1 – Setup (Karate Chop Point)

Tap gently on the side of your hand (the fleshy part under the pinky) while repeating this statement three times:

"Even though I feel stressed and my mind is racing, I deeply and completely accept myself."

The "karate chop point" refers to the fleshy side of your hand, the part you would use to perform a karate chop, located on the outside edge of your hand, below the pinky finger.

This first step sets the tone for the whole process. By naming the issue directly, you bring awareness to what's really happening in the moment, rather than pushing it away.

Step 2 – First Tapping Round (Naming the Stress)

Now tap about 5–7 times on each of the following points while saying the reminder phrase aloud:

- Eyebrow (EB): "This stress"

- Side of Eye (SE): "So much pressure"

- Under Eye (UE): "I feel it in my chest"

- Under Nose (UN): "It's overwhelming"

- Chin (CH): "I can't relax"

- Collarbone (CB): "This stress in my body"

- Under Arm (UA): "I don't know what to do"

- Top of Head (TH): "This stress"

Step 3 – Positive Round (Shifting Into Calm)

Once the intensity starts to ease, repeat the sequence while introducing positive affirmations:

- Eyebrow (EB): "I choose to relax now"

- Side of Eye (SE): "I am safe"

- Under Eye (UE): "I release this stress"

- Under Nose (UN): "I allow peace"

- Chin (CH): "I can handle this"

- Collarbone (CB): "I feel calm"

- Under Arm (UA): "I trust myself"

- Top of Head (TH): "I choose peace now"

Step 4 – Check In

Pause and rate your stress level again on a scale of 0–10.

Repeat another round if needed, until the number drops to a comfortable level.

✦ Variations & Deepening

- **Silent Tapping:** Once you know the sequence, you can just tap silently while feeling the emotion.

- **Body Scan Tapping:** Notice tension in your body and tap while naming the sensation.

- **Affirmation Tapping:** After a stress round, tap with affirmations like "I am worthy," "I am safe," "I allow healing."

- **Quick Fix:** Even just tapping the collarbone point with calm breathing can reduce stress in the moment.

✳ Tips for Best Results

- Always be specific (target one issue at a time).

- Be honest about how you feel (don't jump to positive too fast).

- Repeat rounds until the intensity number drops significantly.

- Consistency matters — a few minutes daily builds stronger results.

- Combine with journaling or meditation for deeper shifts.

21-Day EFT Self-Healing Plan

- **Week 1:** Practice basic EFT once per day on small stresses. Keep a log of intensity before/after.

- **Week 2:** Use EFT for bigger themes (fear, old patterns). Add positive reframes.

- **Week 3:** Create personalized affirmation rounds for goals (confidence, self-love, abundance).

Track progress by writing down shifts in emotion, clarity, or physical ease.

Final Takeaway on EFT

EFT is simple enough to use anywhere, anytime — but powerful enough to change long-standing patterns.

With just your fingertips and a few mindful words, you can calm your nervous system, release stuck energy, and reprogram old beliefs into new ones.

It's free, quick, and portable, one of the most effective self-healing tools you can carry with you for life.

About The Author

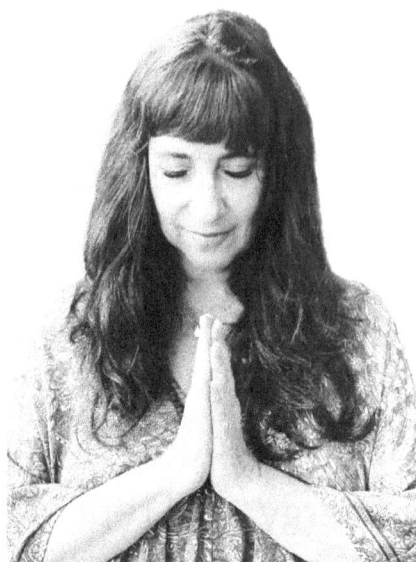

ALLAINE STRICKLEN is a Master Yoga Teacher, Healer, and guide devoted to helping others discover their innate capacity for self-healing. A two-time Brain Surgery survivor, she embodies resilience, and transformation showing that even life's greatest challenges can become gateways to growth. With decades of experience, and a compassionate heart, Allaine inspires others to live with courage, grace and unlimited potential.

Namaste